THE ART OF PARENTING CHILDREN WITH AUTISM AND ASPERGER'S

MEET THEIR UNIQUE NEEDS, SEE THE WORLD THROUGH THEIR EYES, AND UNLOCK THEIR FULL POTENTIAL

AUDRA MILLS

CONTENTS

INTRODUCTION

Every child's behavior is telling us something. Our job is to see the behavior as information, not [frustration].

— UNKNOWN

PEOPLE WITH AUTISM CAN (AND DO) THRIVE

What if I revealed that one of history's most accomplished entrepreneurs is also on the autism spectrum? Would you feel astonished, intrigued, or thrilled? These reactions are quite understandable, considering that many neurodiverse individuals choose to keep their state private to evade discrimination (King, 2022). This stigma, however, was disrupted when the wealthiest man on the planet—who also happens to be the founder of Tesla and SpaceX, a Time Person of the Year, and CEO of Twitter, among other achievements—candidly admitted on live television that he has Asperger's Syndrome (Hargitai et al., 2022).

Elon Musk is merely one of the numerous exceptional individuals who have Autism Spectrum Disorder (ASD). Other noteworthy examples include Eminem, Tim Burton, and Greta Thunberg. ASD is often regarded as "invisible" because people tend to conceal it to avoid prejudice. As a result, Musk's revelation serves a dual purpose: it highlights the significant contributions neurodiverse people provide to society while fostering a sense of empowerment for others with autism (Drake, 2021).

People with ASD are frequently viewed primarily through the lens of their challenges rather than being acknowledged for their extraordinary intellectual abilities. Consequently, the achievements and widespread influence of notable figures such as Elon Musk plays a crucial role in heightening autism awareness and fostering a more thorough understanding of the distinct characteristics associated with this condition—goals that advocates have been tirelessly working towards for a long time.

When influential individuals like Musk share their personal experiences with autism, it helps dispel stereotypes and misconceptions. Doing this paves the way for more inclusivity to recognize the vast potential of people with ASD. In turn, this recognition generates greater opportunities for individuals on the spectrum to thrive, contribute to society, and showcase their unique strengths and talents while also promoting a better understanding of the diverse nature of ASD.

Barriers and Hurdles

Though Elon Musk's success demonstrates that individuals with autism can indeed thrive, it is important to note that his exceptional accomplishments are only one facet and may not be wholly reflective of the broader autistic population (Hargitai et al., 2022). As you and your child navigate life, you will encounter distinct challenges, such as bullying and intolerance. Here are some additional potential obstacles you may be facing:

As a parent, you might experience feelings of helplessness and stress in your daily life as you strive to care for your child with autism. This strain and overwhelming sensation can also impact other areas of your life, including work and relationships.

Being concerned for your child's future is natural. The apprehension of possibly failing as a caregiver, together with the potential feelings of guilt or shame that may be associated with not raising a successful child, can understandably lead to anxiety.

Given the unique stumbling blocks associated with raising a child with ASD, sustaining a healthy and satisfying relationship or marriage becomes even more crucial for the overall emotional well-being of both partners. You know that navigating the complexities of parenting a child with ASD can be a significant source of stress.

There is a desire to confidently attend events or venture out in public without worrying about your child's outbursts or improper conduct. This includes handling unkind individuals and clarifying to family and friends your child's state and expectations.

You seek additional time for personal endeavors, including sufficient rest, moments of tranquility within the household, and the freedom to attend social gatherings independently— all while being reassured that your child and their caregiver are secure in your absence.

You are concerned about the way others interact with your child. There is an underlying fear that they may face bullying, condescending attitudes, and exclusion from social events or interactions. This book offers an approach to helping you and your child with autism achieve their maximum potential while regulating behavior and preserving your well-being as a parent. You have the ability to decrease anxiety and enable them to flourish. By adopting this method, you can take pride in nurturing a thriving, intelligent, and joyful child, inclusive of their neurodiversity. Your child possesses the ability to achieve their full potential, establish meaningful relationships, discover their interests, form friendships, and attain success in adult life. It is also possible for you to accomplish your own goals as a parent and a person.

The Five Pillar Approach

This book presents a Five Pillar approach with strategies that can be applied to problems that come with raising an ASD child and helping them succeed. The pillars do not represent a step-by-step approach that readers must follow sequentially. Instead, they provide a flexible framework that readers can adapt based on the challenges they encounter. Consequently, the book's chapters correspond to individual pillars or a combination thereof without following a strict linear order.

Pillar One: Offers valuable insights to assist you in comprehending the reasons behind the behavior of your child with ASD, enabling you to effectively implement the strategies discussed in Pillar Two below.

Pillar Two: Provides approaches for fostering character growth, unlocking inherent potential, and enhancing abilities, paving the way for success in life.

Pillar Three: Delivers tactics to aid you in handling your child's unpredictable actions, encompassing obsessive and hostile conduct, in addition to addressing sensory challenges.

Pillar Four: Outlines helpful methods to assist you in managing the stress associated with caring for your autistic child while maintaining healthy relationships with your family, despite the challenges that arise in nurturing a child with autism.

Pillar Five: Gives suggestions to assist you in obtaining financial assistance for raising your child with ASD and preparing for their future.

How My Experience Can Benefit You

The inspiration for writing this book stemmed from my involvement in supporting the upbringing of my grandson with Asperger's, aiming to reach out to parents of other children with ASD. I remember one day, when my grandson was six years old, I heard a loud clanking noise from the dining room while I worked in my office. Upon investigating the source of the noise, I discovered the swinging chandelier with its cover plate dislodged from the ceiling. It was at this point that I began to suspect his behavior might extend beyond the realm of typical childhood mischief, leading to his eventual ASD diagnosis.

A profound insight into my grandson's unique perspective occurred during Christmas when he was twelve years old. Together with all of my grandchildren, we visited a neighborhood that displayed extravagant holiday decorations on their homes. However, his favorite house featured only a single illuminated wreath at the peak of its roof. This experience taught me that my grandson cherishes simplicity and has a preference for an uncluttered environment.

At present, he is 24 years old and employed. His progress is evident, especially in the enhancement of his social skills. It has taken me the past two decades to gather the knowledge presented in this book, and I am deeply committed to assisting other families and their children in achieving joyful, harmonious, and prosperous lives. I'd like to demonstrate that neurodiverse children, who may exhibit challenging behaviors in their youth, possess the potential to lead successful lives in the future.

Navigating the path to adequately support my grandson in achieving his fullest potential was challenging for our family due to the lack of information we previously had. The insights presented here aim to enhance your understanding of your child's actions. Learning from these lessons may help reduce anxiety and strengthen your confidence in the path to independence for your child. This way, you can all participate socially with assurance and tackle any queries others may have about your child. By lowering the stress in your life, it is possible to regain control over your professional and personal relationships, including those with existing or potential partners. Now is the time to rediscover personal time and bring peace back into your home. You are the perfect parent to help your child thrive.

1

WHAT YOU NEED TO KNOW ABOUT AUTISM SPECTRUM DISORDER (ASD) AND ASPERGER'S SYNDROME

In a dark place we find ourselves, and a little more knowledge lights our way.

— YODA

WHAT IS AUTISM SPECTRUM DISORDER (ASD)?

This chapter corresponds to Pillar One of the Five Pillar Approach and will give you more information about Autism Spectrum Disorder (ASD) and Asperger's in order to better understand your child's condition. Understanding the subtleties of ASD can provide insight into the fact that the experiences of ASD are unique to each individual. There is no one-size-fits-all label.

Autism is considered a "spectrum" because its symptoms and severity vary greatly among affected individuals. It is defined as a developmental (sometimes neurological) disorder impacting communication, social interaction, learning abilities, and behavior. While individuals can be diagnosed at any age, it is referred to as a "developmental disorder" because symptoms generally occur in the first two years of life (National Institute of Mental Health, 2022).

Signs and Symptoms

Individuals with ASD struggle with communication, both verbal and non-verbal, and may have difficulty interpreting social cues and forming friendships, which can lead to feelings of isolation. Repetitive behaviors and sensory sensitivities can also disrupt their daily lives. Each person with autism is unique, and support and understanding are essential for them to thrive. Developmental monitoring can help detect early signs of ASD, which typically become consistently observable by age two or three (CDC, 2019a). Children with ASD may exhibit some, but not all, of the following behaviors.

Social Communication and Interaction Behaviors

According to the National Institute of Mental Health (2022), individuals with ASD commonly exhibit some social communication and interaction behaviors, which include:

- Refraining from making or maintaining regular eye contact
- Appearing disinterested, unresponsive, or unaware when conversing with others
- Rarely expressing enthusiasm, affection, or pleasure for items or activities (including showing or pointing at things to others)
- Failing to respond or having a delayed response time to one's name or to other verbal invitations for attention
- Encountering challenges with the give-and-take of conversation
- Talking passionately about a favorite subject for long periods without recognizing that others may not be interested or without allowing others to participate
- Displaying facial movements, gestures, and expressions that do not coincide with the words being spoken
- Using an abnormal tone of voice that may sound monotonous or robotic-like
- Finding it challenging to comprehend another's perspective or having difficulty predicting or understanding the behavior of others
- Encountering problems with adapting behaviors to social surroundings
- Difficulties participating in imaginative play or forming friendships.

Restricted or Repetitive Behaviors or Interests

As per the CDC, individuals with ASD may exhibit atypical behaviors or have interests that can be considered unusual (2019a). These particular behaviors and interests differentiate from other conditions characterized only by difficulties with social communication and interaction:

- Arranging toys or objects in a particular way and becoming upset if that order is altered
- Repeating words or phrases (known as echolalia)
- Engaging in the same play behaviors every time
- Focusing intently on certain parts of objects (such as wheels)
- Reacting negatively to even minor changes
- Having fixations or obsessions
- Following specific routines
- Making repetitive movements such as rocking, spinning, or flapping hands
- Having unusual reactions to sensory stimuli such as sounds, smells, tastes, appearances, or textures
- Being more or less sensitive to sensory inputs such as light, sound, clothing, food, or temperature.

What Causes ASD?

The specific cause of ASD remains unknown, but it is linked to differences in the brain. Some people have a genetic condition that contributes to ASD, while other factors are yet to be identified. Research suggests that gene-environment interactions can impact development, leading to ASD. Having an older parent, a sibling with ASD, a very low birth weight, or certain genetic conditions can increase the likelihood of developing ASD (National Institute of Mental Health, 2022). There are certain medications, like valproic acid and thalidomide, that have been associated with an increased risk of autism when taken during pregnancy (Dietert et al., 2011). Pregnant women taking these medications should be aware of the potential risks to their unborn child. It is important to discuss any medication use during pregnancy with a healthcare provider to ensure the safety and health of both the mother and baby. Several studies have revealed that individuals with ASD have notable increases in mercury biomarkers, suggesting mercury poisoning (Voight, n.d.). We still have much to learn about the influence of these factors on individuals with ASD.

Diagnosis

ASD diagnosis requires a comprehensive evaluation of behavior and developmental milestones by a team of medical experts. Diagnosis relies on comparing behavior to established criteria since there are no definitive medical tests for ASD. The team typically consists of psychiatrists, psychologists, neurologists, and developmental pediatricians who will evaluate language skills, social behavior, and cognitive abilities, and may use additional assessments. Early diagnosis is crucial for early intervention to impact development and social adjustment.

In Young Children

The process of diagnosis in young children usually involves two stages: The first is a general developmental screening that takes place during regular checkups, and the second is an additional diagnostic evaluation.

Stage 1: Developmental Screening

Regular checkups with a pediatrician or early childhood healthcare provider are important for all children. During these appointments, developmental delays, including ASD screenings at 18 and 24 months, will be assessed. Additional screening may be necessary if there is a higher likelihood of ASD. Caregiver concerns are also taken into account during the screening process. The doctor may ask about the child's behavior and combine that with information from ASD screening tools and clinical observations. If developmental differences are detected during screening, the child may be referred for further evaluation.

Stage 2: Developmental Diagnosis

If a screening tool indicates an area of concern, a developmental evaluation may be needed to accurately identify a child's strengths and challenges with ASD. Trained specialists will assess the child's behavior, cognitive and language abilities, and daily activities. A detailed discussion with caregivers will also take place. The evaluation can determine if the child meets the requirements for a developmental diagnosis, and treatment recommendations can be made accordingly.

In Older Children and Adolescents

Teachers are typically the first to recognize ASD symptoms in older children and adolescents attending school. The school's special education team may conduct an initial assessment and recommend further evaluation by a primary healthcare provider or an ASD specialist (National Institute of Mental Health, 2022). Socializing with peers can be challenging for children on the spectrum due to difficulties in understanding tone, facial expressions, body language, figures of speech, jokes, or sarcasm. Caregivers can discuss their child's social difficulties with healthcare providers.

In Adults

Increased awareness of ASD has led to more adults seeking assessments later in life. However, this can be complicated by overlapping symptoms with other mental health disorders and the development of coping mechanisms (Beversdorf, 2014). Diagnostic techniques used for children can be applied to adults, and your doctors can provide referrals. During the evaluation, experts will ask about issues related to sensory processing, repetitive behaviors, social communication, and interaction. An adult diagnosis can provide insight into past difficulties, current strengths, and appropriate services and support (National Institute of Mental Health, 2022).

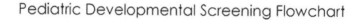

Pediatric Developmental Screening Flowchart

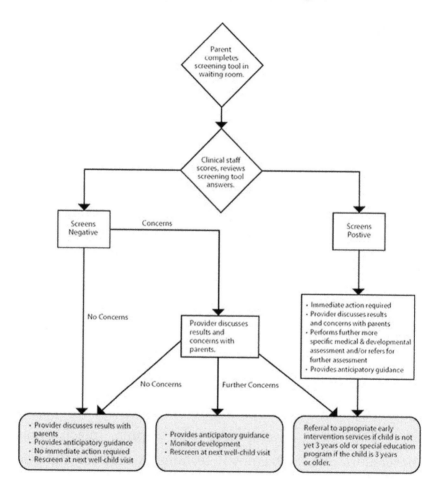

Treatment and Therapies

ASD cannot be cured, but it offers a unique perspective on the world. There is a debate between two groups: one sees it as a disability that requires medical intervention, while the other prioritizes securing disability rights such as equitable employment practices and healthcare coverage (Jewell, 2020). Nonetheless, being on the spectrum can present challenges, and appropriate care can help individuals develop their strengths and acquire new skills.

Medication

There is no medication to treat ASD. However, a child psychiatrist, in conjunction with the child's parents, may prescribe medication to address symptoms such as hyperactivity, aggression, irritability, repetitive behavior, anxiety, and depression. Although there is no supplement that can cure autism, certain supplements such as multivitamins and minerals, melatonin, probiotics, N-acetylcysteine (NAC), L-carnosine, L-carnitine, Ubiquinol, Omega-3 fatty acids, Vitamin D, and Vitamin C may help reduce specific symptoms (Cooperman, n.d.). The adaptogenic properties of ashwagandha may also prove beneficial (Vijayalakshmi & Kripa, 2015).

Behavioral, Psychological, and Educational Interventions

Behavioral

Behavioral approaches, including applied behavioral analysis (ABA), are effective in treating ASD symptoms. ABA involves analyzing challenges and designing a plan to improve adaptive skills and decrease inappropriate behavior (CDC, 2019b). Two styles of ABA teaching are Discrete Trial Training (DTT) and Pivotal Response Training (PRT). DTT breaks lessons down into simple parts with step-by-step instructions, while PRT aims to improve pivotal skills in a natural setting.

Psychological

CBT is an effective psychological intervention for managing mental health challenges such as anxiety or depression in individuals with ASD. It explores the connections between thoughts, emotions, and behavior with the goal of modifying problematic thought processes through collaborative work between the individual with ASD and their therapist. By changing how they respond to situations, individuals can learn to better manage their mental health and cope with daily life challenges, leading to improved self-awareness, emotional regulation, and social functioning.

Educational

The TEACCH method is an educational intervention for individuals with ASD that emphasizes structured learning environments and visual aids (CDC, 2019b). Educators can customize the classroom arrangement and enhance academic outcomes by using techniques such as displaying daily routines in written or pictorial formats, creating defined learning areas, and supplementing spoken instructions with visual or physical demonstrations.

When to See a Doctor

Early intervention is crucial for the successful treatment of Autism Spectrum Disorder (ASD). Contact your child's doctor if you suspect they may have ASD, as early detection greatly increases the chances for positive outcomes in learning, communication, and behavior. Early identification of ASD can also set your child up for long-term well-being. Be aware of key indicators of ASD, such as delays in communication and social interaction, which usually manifest in the first few years of a child's life. Seek the help of a trained and qualified professional for a comprehensive assessment if you notice any of these symptoms.

DISPROVING MYTHS ABOUT AUTISM

Autism is often misunderstood due to pervasive myths and untruths. These misconceptions arise from a lack of understanding and experience with autism. Stereotypes perpetuated by media and entertainment harm children with autism and their families. Here are eight common misunderstandings and the truth behind them.

ASD Causes Intellectual Disabilities

People with autism can achieve higher education and successful careers in different fields. However, standardized IQ tests may not accurately measure their unique intellectual abilities.

People With ASD Lack Empathy

Individuals with autism experience emotions and may have heightened empathy, but their expression of emotions may not always be immediately recognizable due to anxiety or difficulty demonstrating empathy in a conventional manner.

ASD Is Caused by the Environment

Autism is largely believed to be genetic, with twin studies indicating a 90% chance of the other twin also having ASD and parents of a child with ASD being more likely to have a second child with ASD (Tick et al., 2016).

Girls Don't Get ASD

ASD is more common in boys with a 4:1 ratio, but it is still present in girls. Girls are more likely to be misdiagnosed, while boys are more likely to be diagnosed at birth (Novak, 2022). ASD has a genetic component and tends to run in families.

ASD Is the Same for Everyone

ASD is a complex condition with varying symptoms and challenges. The cause of the differences in the brains of those with ASD is not fully understood, and no two people with ASD will have identical life experiences due to the diverse nature of the disorder.

Vaccines Cause Autism

The link between vaccines and ASD is a widely discredited myth. The idea originated from a retracted study published in The Lancet, and there is no scientific evidence to support this claim.

ASD Can Be Cured

Early behavioral treatment can help individuals with ASD develop the necessary adaptive skills for everyday life, including emotional and behavioral regulation and social engagement, despite the lack of a known cure.

People With ASD Have Special Skills

People with ASD have strengths and weaknesses like everyone else, and being on the spectrum does not guarantee exceptional abilities. However, some individuals may exhibit above-average skills in certain areas compared to their general abilities.

DIFFERENCES AND SIMILARITIES BETWEEN AUTISM AND ASPERGERS

Previously, we have discussed ASD broadly. However, it is important to focus on Asperger's Syndrome specifically. While it falls within the wider range of spectrum disorders, Asperger's has unique defining characteristics that distinguish it from other forms of ASD.

Asperger's vs. Autism

Previously, Asperger's syndrome and ASD were regarded as distinct and separate conditions. The differences between them were discovered by Dr. Lorna Wing, a British psychiatrist who translated the work of Hans Asperger, an Austrian physician. Asperger's identified unique characteristics in autistic children with milder symptoms, but as of 2013, Asperger's is now considered part of the autism spectrum and is no longer diagnosed separately. Some individuals may still identify with Asperger's, as it forms part of their self-concept. The only notable difference between ASD and Asperger's is that individuals with Asperger's may find it easier to pass as neurotypical with fewer signs and symptoms. Furthermore, Asperger's syndrome is less associated with language delays and may lead to a later diagnosis.

Diagnostic Criteria for Asperger's Syndrome

The Diagnostic and Statistical Manual of Mental Disorders (DSM) is a widely used handbook containing descriptions, symptoms, and other criteria for use in diagnosing mental disorders. Asperger's diagnosis criteria were previously in the DSM-IV, which has since been updated to the DSM-5. You can compare this list to the signs and symptoms of social communication and interaction behaviors and restricted or repetitive behaviors or interests for ASD earlier in this chapter.

- Difficulty in verbal or nonverbal communication, such as avoiding eye contact or understanding sarcasm
- Having limited or no long-term social connections with peers
- No enthusiasm for participating in social activities or engaging in shared interests with others
- Exhibiting minimal or negligible reaction towards social or emotional situations
- Maintaining a prolonged fascination with one specific subject or only a small number of subjects
- Maintaining a strong commitment to carrying out habitual or routine actions consistently
- Repetitive actions or movements that are done over and over again
- High level of curiosity directed towards particular features of objects
- Difficulty maintaining relationships, jobs, or other aspects of daily life because of their symptoms
- Not experiencing any delays in language learning or cognitive development that are commonly observed in other neurodevelopmental disorders with similar symptoms (Jewell, 2020).

Treatment Options

Psychological Therapy

Asperger's Syndrome can create communication and inter-action challenges, but therapy and treatment can help individuals find success. Early intervention is crucial for beneficial outcomes. Cognitive behavioral therapy can address concurrent anxiety or depression. Social skills training improves communication skills and understanding of social cues. Physical or occupational therapy focuses on improving movement and coordination skills. Family therapy involves the entire family in the therapeutic process to promote good social and living skills. ABA can improve social and communication skills in children with Asperger's by promoting positive behavior and discouraging negative behavior. The type of ABA therapy used may vary based on age and targeted skill areas.

Medications

No approved medications exist for treating Asperger's or ASD, but medication may be prescribed for coexisting conditions such as anxiety, OCD, depression, ADHD, bipolar disorder, and sleep problems. Antidepressants like SSRIs can be used for anxiety and depression, while drugs like methylphenidate are used for ADHD. Mood stabilizers, antipsychotics, and antidepressants can be used for bipolar disorder, and melatonin supplements can help with sleep problems.

Speech and Language Therapy

Speech and language therapy can benefit individuals with Asperger's Syndrome, despite their typically strong language abilities. This therapy can help improve conversational tone and the ability to perceive and respond to figurative language. It can also help individuals with Asperger's recognize nuances in language and develop effective communication strategies, leading to improved social interactions and communication skills.

Art and Music Therapy

Art and music therapy use creative activities like drawing, painting, music, and singing to address different needs. They are particularly effective at improving communication and social skills. For instance, those engaging in music-making with others develop behaviors like eye contact, taking turns, and active engagement with another person (Seladi-Schulman, 2019). By providing a non-judgmental environment for expression, individuals can build self-awareness and self-esteem, and explore new coping mechanisms. Art and music therapy also treat depression and anxiety. They engage both cognitive and emotional faculties for a holistic approach.

Diet

People with ASD may try dietary treatments, such as a gluten-free or casein-free diet, as part of their symptom management. While some individuals report benefits, there is no conclusive evidence on the efficacy of such diets for Asperger's (Seladi-Schulman, 2019). Additionally, those with ASD may have difficulty with certain foods or limited diets, so it is important to consult with medical and nutrition professionals. A personalized and flexible approach is recommended.

Lack of Treatment

Untreated Asperger's can have a significant impact on a child's development and well-being. Children with Asperger's may struggle with instructions, social communication, and fine motor skills. They may also have difficulty managing a full school day and participating in athletic activities, leading to a sedentary lifestyle and an increased risk for obesity and other health issues. Low self-esteem, bullying, and social isolation can also be challenges. Developing social communication skills, managing anxiety and stress, and coping with academic expectations can all contribute to a complex set of hurdles for children with Asperger's.

Similarities

ASD and Asperger's syndrome have some differences, but they share many commonalities in terms of their symptoms. Children with either condition can find it challenging to maintain relationships and have difficulty expressing their feelings or emotions. Maintaining eye contact may be arduous, and they could have sensitivities to specific foods or sounds. Problems with motor skills are common, and they might have a strong desire to follow rigid schedules. Children with these conditions likely also obsess over specific topics.

Individuals with both ASD and Asperger's can be seen as socially awkward by others, and hand-flapping is a common behavior in those with either disorder. These conditions often require specialized support and care to help individuals lead productive and fulfilling lives. It is meaningful to get an accurate diagnosis in order to create a tailored treatment plan that meets the individual's unique needs. With the right support, people with autism and Asperger's can thrive and develop strong relationships with those around them.

RAISING A CHILD WITH ASPERGER'S

Recently, a friend of mine learned that her son has ASD. Although this news undoubtedly presented a challenge for the family, I was glad to see that they were accepting the diagnosis with a positive attitude and without overreacting.

Evan's Diagnosis

As a first-time mother, it was challenging to anticipate my son Evan's actions. He never seemed to enjoy socializing with other children during our toddler activity classes, preferring to stay close to me. Although we lived in a family-friendly neighborhood with a lot of other youngsters around the same age, he found parks particularly disturbing because of the high noise levels. It troubled me the most that he seemed disinclined to communicate with my husband and me, although he could speak.

Evan adored cars and spent hours sorting his toys into an ordered arrangement. At clean-up time, he would become agitated. He had trouble grasping pencils and was unable to draw or trace a line or circle, a skill I thought would develop more during preschool. However, when preschool eventually arrived, Evan was hardly enthusiastic about attending.

When the pandemic broke out soon afterward, Evan became agitated when he had to stay at home rather than go to school. He struggled to understand why we couldn't go to school after breakfast and brushing our teeth. The only thing that could soothe him was sitting by the window and watching vehicles drive by. He fidgeted constantly with his fingers, flicking them repeatedly.

When I discussed this behavior with my own therapist, she suggested that I contact a pediatrician. We were eventually able to arrange a telehealth developmental assessment with a practitioner who could observe Evan in his natural environment with his toys. The diagnosis of ASD was suggested since Evan exhibited several symptoms, not just a few.

I have learned that Evan perceives the world differently than most people, and we have tried to support him and see things from his perspective. He has started working with a speech and language therapist and has begun to open up a little more. During a stroll with him, we spotted a bird perched on a nearby fence. Evan excitedly pointed at the bird and said, "Mommy, look!" Some individuals may regard this as a small, insignificant moment, but for us, it was a breakthrough. Sometimes, it's the tiniest advancements that make the greatest impact.

Celebrities

Celebrities sharing their personal stories of raising children on the autism spectrum can help reduce stigma and promote acceptance of ASD. Their public platform allows them to amplify the voices of the autism community and advocate for the support and resources needed to thrive.

Sylvester Stallone

Sylvester Stallone's son was diagnosed with ASD at age 3, prompting him to film a PSA commercial in 1990 to raise awareness. He continues to use his fame to advocate for ASD research and awareness.

Tommy Hilfiger

Tommy Hilfiger, a well-known designer, created a PSA for Autism Speaks to honor his daughter, who was diagnosed with autism at age five. He emphasizes the importance of early intervention and wishes more people cared about autism due to the lack of research and funding. Hilfiger became an advocate and designed a successful clothing line for individuals with ASD, including adults. His daughter, who is highly intelligent, is comforted by her neurodivergent stepbrother.

Toni Braxton

Toni Braxton, a Grammy-award winning singer, has publicly shared her experience with her son's autism diagnosis, and largely attributes his remarkable progress to early intervention and the resources provided by Autism Speaks. She encourages others to approach autism with an open mind and view it as simply a different way of learning, rather than a deficiency. Toni's son, now 18 years old, has achieved success as a model in the fashion industry, and she encourages other parents to seek out the assistance they need to help their children thrive.

KEY POINTS AND TAKEAWAYS

In this chapter, we covered a lot of ground on ASD to help you better support your child, aligning with Pillar One of the Five Pillar approach. We discussed signs, symptoms, diagnosis, treatment, and common myths about ASD. We also explored Asperger's syndrome and shared personal stories from celebrity parents and a friend of the author. Next, we will focus on coping with stress and maintaining healthy relationships while caring for a child with ASD. We will provide strategies for managing stress and guidance on informing family members and loved ones about your child's diagnosis.

2

TELLING YOUR LOVED ONES AND OTHER PEOPLE ABOUT THE DIAGNOSIS

Even for parents of children that are not on the spectrum, there is no such thing as a normal child.

— VIOLET STEVENS

ON YOUR TERMS

This section is related to Pillar Four of the Five Pillar approach. The fourth pillar provides a comprehensive set of helpful methods to manage the stress that inevitably comes with being a parent of a neurodivergent child. It also delves into maintaining positive relationships with your family despite the various challenges you may face while nurturing and raising a child with ASD. Additionally, it involves finding effective ways to ensure that you can devote sufficient time and attention to your emotional, mental, and physical health.

Telling Others Your Child Has ASD

Discussing your child's autism diagnosis with others can be a difficult task. It's natural to feel hesitant about disclosing this information and worry about how others may react or treat your child. However, it's important to remember that autism is a genetic neurological condition, and there is nothing to be ashamed of. Educating others about your child's needs and behavior can help them understand how to interact with your child and dispel any misconceptions about autism. Planning the conversation ahead of time and choosing a private and comfortable setting can also help. Be prepared to answer any questions that may arise, and remember that your love and support are crucial to your child's well-being. By sharing information about autism, you can increase understanding and acceptance of neurodiversity.

When to Tell People

Deciding when to share your child's ASD diagnosis is a personal and difficult decision. It's important to consider your own feelings and needs before disclosing it to others. Remember that you are your child's best advocate and should always feel empowered to make decisions in their best interest. Take your time and decide when the right time is for you and your family.

Tip

There are ways to handle challenging situations where your child's behavior is misunderstood without revealing their diagnosis. Excusing yourself politely and taking your child to a private space to regroup can help you tend to their needs while respecting their privacy; e.g., saying, "Please excuse us, we need to go to another room to calm down for a moment" (Beaming Health, 2023) can be an effective strategy.

When Is the Right Time

It's important to remember that you're not obligated to disclose your child's ASD diagnosis unless necessary. You can choose to share it when you feel ready, rather than under pressure or stress, to avoid feeling frustrated with your delivery. Being well-informed and empowered is important, so waiting until you have a thorough understanding of your child's condition is recommended. Choosing the right setting is also vital; a private, relaxed, and neutral environment with enough time and space to answer questions and establish boundaries is ideal. Additionally, consider your loved ones' familiarity with children on the spectrum and provide resources or further information as necessary. Planning and preparing the conversation can lead to a more productive outcome. If you're not in the right state of mind to engage in the conversation, it's wise to regroup and try again later.

Tip

Anticipate that discussing your child's diagnosis with family members may result in difficult reactions, which can vary greatly from person to person. These responses may include feelings of relief, sadness, or even rejection. It is important to give your family members space to express their emotions, even if they differ from your own. While it is normal for a range of emotions to occur, it is important to remember that these reactions may leave you feeling hurt or isolated.

If There Isn't a Right Time

Sharing your child's autism diagnosis with others may become necessary at times, even if it's not in an ideal or comfortable environment. If you think it could benefit your child by helping others understand them better, or if it's necessary to manage unrealistic expectations of your child's behavior or abilities, consider sharing. While it can be challenging to share such personal information, remember that you are simply advocating for your child's needs, and you don't owe anyone an explanation.

Sharing your child's ASD diagnosis can be especially helpful in situations where they are experiencing distress or difficulty. A brief explanation that your child is on the spectrum can help reduce stress and tension in these situations. Additionally, correcting unrealistic expectations can help reduce stress for your child and educate others about the realities of ASD. As a parent, you may know certain tasks or situations that are difficult for your child, and you can speak up in those situations to correct these unrealistic expectations.

Ultimately, sharing your child's diagnosis is a personal decision, and you should only share when you feel it's necessary or beneficial. However, remember that you are your child's best advocate and that any reasonable person will understand and offer support.

Tip

At a neighborhood barbecue, if your child hits another kid and someone else you know believes you need to discipline your child better, you can explain to the other parent that your child is on the autism spectrum and struggles with being gentle. Alternatively, you can explain to the acquaintance that your child has ASD and becomes overwhelmed in social situations and needs a break, and that their behavior is not intentional misbehavior that requires punishment.

How to Tell People

To effectively explain your child's ASD diagnosis to others, consider using visual aids such as videos, picture books, and infographics. These tools can simplify the complexities of ASD and make them more understandable. It's also important to use clear and concise language, especially when speaking to someone who is not familiar with autism.

To personalize your child's diagnosis, use specific examples from their daily life to illustrate their strengths and challenges. This will help others understand how ASD impacts their lives in unique ways. It's essential for others to recognize that autism is a permanent part of your child's identity, and that it both contributes to their strengths and presents challenges.

As the expert on your child and their disorder, you can use your own experiences and observations to help others understand what ASD means for your family. While explanations of ASD can be complex and medical, sharing your knowledge and advocating for your child can help others appreciate the richness and complexity of neurodiverse experiences.

Tip

Focus on the basics of what autism entails, such as the fact that it is a genetic neurodevelopmental disorder that begins in utero and is not caused by vaccines or bad parenting.

TIPS FOR SHARING

Prioritize your child's needs and well-being when sharing their autism diagnosis. Though challenging, it can provide support for them to thrive. Different groups may need different approaches, such as educating family members and outlining accommodations for school officials.

Emphasize your child's strengths to reduce the stigma surrounding ASD. Involve your child in the decision about who to share the diagnosis with. Sharing the diagnosis can be difficult, but it's necessary for their well-being. Approach it with care, sensitivity, and positivity to help others understand and support your child's growth.

Loved Ones

When discussing your child's needs with family members or loved ones, choose a time when you feel alert and ready to have the conversation. Make sure you're in a relaxed and comfortable setting for both you and the other individual. Do your research beforehand and try to understand as much as possible about your child's strengths and weaknesses. If needed, utilize visual aids such as videos or infographics to help explain difficult concepts. Try to draw from your child's personal experiences and provide examples to help clarify and simplify the information for your loved ones.

Siblings

It's important to start this conversation early on, as children may begin to notice their siblings' differences and have questions. Picture books can serve as a helpful visual aid to explain the concept of autism in a way that children can understand.

When introducing these books, it's important to use simple language and concepts that are appropriate for their age. You can use the book to explain that their sibling's brain works a little differently and that they may struggle with certain things that other children find easy. It's also important to emphasize that their sibling is still the same person they love, and that their differences don't make them any less lovable.

Some great picture books that can help explain autism to younger siblings include "My Brother Charlie" by Holly Robinson Peete and Ryan Elizabeth Peete, "The Autism Acceptance Book" by Ellen Sabin, and "All My Stripes: A Story for Children with Autism" by Shaina Rudolph and Danielle Royer. By using these resources and having open and honest conversations, you can help your children better understand their sibling's autism and foster a positive and accepting relationship between them.

Law Enforcement Officers

When speaking to law enforcement, it's important to communicate in a clear and concise manner. Here are some tips if you find yourself in a situation where you need to interact with law enforcement: Stick to sharing short, factual statements about your child's behavior. To avoid confusion, it can also be helpful for your child to wear a medical alert bracelet or other visible identifier. This can prevent police from mistaking your child's reaching for a communication device or ID as reaching for a weapon. Additionally, you may want to consider using "Autistic child on board" stickers on your vehicle. This could be particularly useful in a situation where you need quick and clear communication during an emergency. Taking these steps can help ensure that law enforcement responds in a more informed and appropriate manner when interacting with your child.

Strangers

If you find yourself in a public space and your child with autism is experiencing a meltdown, it can be helpful to use straightforward and clear communication with strangers to help explain the situation. You can use simple language to describe that your child has ASD, which can help others understand why they may be behaving differently than what is considered typical. Additionally, it can be useful to provide accurate and factual information related to the behavior and needs of individuals with autism, countering any misconceptions or assumptions that strangers may have. Remember, explanations don't need to be overly complex or lengthy, but rather concise and informative to help others better comprehend and respond to your child's behavior.

Uninformed or Judgmental People

When someone makes inaccurate or critical comments about autism or your child's behavior, it's important to advocate for your child. Use factual, straightforward language to correct people when necessary. For example, if someone implies that your child's autism diagnosis is something to be pitied, you could say something like, "Actually, autism is a neurological difference that's part of what makes my child unique. I'm proud of them and everything they bring to the world" (Beaming Health, 2023). It's also important to challenge misconceptions about autism, such as the belief that it exists on a linear scale. Remind people that autism is a complex and diverse spectrum, with each person having their own challenges and strengths. By speaking up with kindness and clarity, you can help create a more inclusive and compassionate world for everyone.

Children

Explaining ASD to young children can be challenging. It is important to use language that is appropriate for their age and to encourage them to ask questions without being shamed. Ignoring the subject and treating it as taboo can lead to confusion and misunderstandings.

One effective approach is to emphasize the importance of manners and empathy. Helping children understand that individuals with autism are not behaving badly but are trying to manage something that is difficult for them can foster compassion and understanding. Encourage children to ask questions and have open discussions about their thoughts and feelings.

When choosing picture books to guide the conversation, ensure that the story mirrors the child's experience. Reading about a child with autism who is nonverbal and flaps their hands may not resonate with a child whose friend with autism is highly verbal and social (Loiselle, 2021). By providing accurate information and creating a safe space for discussion, children can develop a better understanding of

ASD and learn to appreciate and accept individual differences.

IF YOUR FAMILY IS NOT RECEPTIVE

Not everyone in your circle may be supportive of your child's autism diagnosis. Dealing with those who deny or view autism negatively can be frustrating. However, it's better to address their concerns with factual and under-standable language. Educating these individuals about autism can make a significant difference, but it may require them to learn new knowledge and skills. To help them understand, it could be useful to use analogies such as, "Just like you wouldn't punish a blind person for bumping into something because it's beyond their control, autism also presents challenges that require a different type of support" (Beaming Health, 2023).

It's essential to communicate clear boundaries with loved ones and acquaintances who may not understand the impacts of autism. If they are unwilling to adjust their actions or expectations, it's crucial to firmly communicate what you will do, including the consequences. By doing so, you are protecting your child and ensuring that they receive the necessary support and care.

SETTING BOUNDARIES WITH LOVED ONES

It's important to set boundaries with people who may not be supportive of your child's autism diagnosis, even if they are family or close friends. Sometimes, loved ones may have expectations or behaviors that can harm your child's growth and development, and it's necessary to take action to protect them. As a parent, you are your child's best advocate and protector, so it's important to treat this situation like any other that could potentially harm your child. Remember that your child's well-being should always be a priority, and don't be afraid to set boundaries with those who may not understand or support your child's needs. This could mean having difficult conversations, reducing communication or contact, or seeking outside support from professionals or support groups. By setting clear boundaries, you can create a safer and more supportive environment for your child to grow and thrive in.

IF YOU AND YOUR PARTNER DISAGREE

If you find yourself in a situation where you and your partner or co-parent are not in agreement about your child's ASD diagnosis, it can be incredibly stressful for everyone involved. It's essential to try to work together and come to a shared understanding of what your child needs. One way to do this is by seeking knowledge from experts and other parents. Take the time to gather information, read up on the subject, and discuss it together. If your partner or co-parent is resistant, there may be a larger communication issue that needs to be addressed.

It's also critical to prioritize maintaining your relationship. There may have been underlying issues in your relationship that existed before your child's diagnosis, and it's important not to neglect those. Keeping your relationship healthy and loving will make it easier to come to a resolution about your differing opinions. Take time to spend together, whether it's going on dates or simply having a conversation over dinner. Seek out couples therapy or individual therapy, if necessary, to work through any issues that may be impacting your relationship. Remember, you're on the same team, and you both want what's best for your child. By working together and prioritizing your relationship, you can find a way to support your child and each other.

EXPLAINING YOUR CHILD'S CARE

When it comes to sharing information about your child's ASD with friends and family, it's important to strike a balance between what they need to know and what they don't. However, if these individuals are involved in caring for your child, there may be certain things that they need to be aware of to ensure a successful and positive experience.

For example, if your child doesn't like physical touch, it's important to let others know that hugs or other forms of physical affection may not be appreciated. Similarly, if your child has any dietary restrictions, it's important to make those known to anyone who may be offering them food. Establishing routines and setting expectations can also be incredibly beneficial to children with autism, as unexpected events or changes to the routine can be particularly upsetting.

While it's important to provide guidance and information to friends and family members caring for your child, it's also necessary to remember that not all behaviors or challenges require punishment. Sometimes, disruptions to routines or unexpected behavior can be particularly overwhelming for children with autism, and it's important to approach these situations with understanding and patience.

Additionally, it's important to help friends and family members understand the specific goals for your child. For example, if you are working on maintaining eye contact during conversation, it may be helpful to explain this goal to those interacting with you. With the right guidance and support, friends and family members can play an important role in helping children on the spectrum thrive.

KEY POINTS AND TAKEAWAYS

The aim of this chapter was to provide you with practical strategies to inform your loved ones and others about your child's diagnosis of ASD, in line with Pillar Four of the Five

Pillar approach, which focuses on managing the stress of caring for your child with autism while maintaining healthy relationships with your family. Although there is no perfect time to disclose your child's condition, we suggest striving towards ideal conditions, such as when you are relaxed, informed, and have ample energy. If your child's ASD is causing them distress or someone has unrealistic expectations of them, speaking up can help reduce stress and educate others.

We also provide resources such as videos, picture books, and infographics to aid in communicating with family members, siblings, law enforcement officers, and strangers, as well as suggestions for preparing for conversations with those who may not be receptive to your child's diagnosis. Setting boundaries with judgmental or uninformed family members, partners, or strangers is crucial to minimizing stress and cultivating supportive relationships.

Moving forward, the next chapter will focus on how children with ASD communicate, and we will provide strategies for parents to communicate effectively with their children while empowering them to interact with others. This aligns with Pillar Two of the Five Pillar framework, which aims to build your child's character, discover their potential, and enhance their skills to support them in achieving success in life.

3

HELPING THEM DEVELOP COMMUNICATION SKILLS

Yesterday is not ours to recover, but tomorrow is ours to win or lose.

— LYNDON B. JOHNSON

MAKING CONNECTIONS

This section explores effective strategies for parents to communicate with their autistic children and facilitate their interactions with others. It aligns with Pillar Two of the Five Pillar framework, which emphasizes practical techniques to enable parents to support their child's character development, identify their strengths, and help them enhance their skills to build confidence and thrive in life. To facilitate communication, it's important to use simple language and visual aids, be patient, and give them space and time to process and respond. Encouragement and positive feedback can motivate them to continue building their skills, and seeking professional help is recommended if needed. Structured settings and technology can also be useful in developing social communication skills. With patience and support, you can help your child communicate and interact more effectively with others.

HOW AUTISTIC CHILDREN COMMUNICATE

Communication skills are crucial for all children. Autistic children have varying communication abilities, with some having language delays or difficulties expressing themselves verbally. It's important to provide them with support to learn and practice their skills. They may communicate differently, incorporating non-verbal communication and behavior to express themselves. Working on communication together can improve your relationship and help them communicate better with others.

Language

Echolalia is a common communication behavior observed in autistic children, where they repeat words or phrases heard from others, videos, or TV shows. This repetition often lacks context and can be expressed in an unusual tone. In addition, they may create new words, repeat the same word multiple times, or struggle with pronouns, such as mixing up "I" and "you."

It is essential to recognize that these behaviors are an attempt to communicate, even though they may be challenging for others to interpret. Autistic children may learn language by repeating phrases associated with specific emotional states or situations, and then deducing their meanings by observing their effects. Therefore, they may say, "Do you want some chocolate?" when they really want chocolate themselves because they associate the phrase with receiving chocolate in the past (Raising Children Network Australia, 2021).

Nonverbal Communication

Autistic children may use physical actions to guide a person or object, such as pushing a person's hand towards something they desire. They may also indicate what they want or need by pointing, showing, or shifting their gaze. Additionally, using objects can be a part of nonverbal communication, such as handing an object to someone as a way of communicating.

Behavior

Children who are neurodivergent may exhibit challenging behavior, which is often linked to communication difficulties. Such behavior includes self-harm, outbursts, and aggression towards others. It is the child's way of expressing their needs, unhappiness, confusion, or fear.

As a parent, it is essential to understand your child's perspective to interpret the message behind their behavior. Try to analyze the situation and interpret their behavior to address their needs accurately.

COMMUNICATION STRATEGIES

Language impairment is a common characteristic of autism, which can make it challenging for children to express themselves and comprehend what others are saying. This can lead to misunderstandings, with adults often mistaking the child's difficulties for disobedience. It can be likened to being in a foreign country where the language is unfamiliar, making it impossible to respond to calls in that language. To support your child's language and communication skills, autism communication strategies can be implemented. Speech therapists are experts who can evaluate language development, provide guidance on intervention planning, and recommend effective strategies. ABA therapy, which uses positive reinforcement techniques, has also been shown to improve communication abilities. There are several books about ABA Visual Language that can help parents.

Visual Supports

Visual supports are tools that use symbols, photos, written words, and objects to help children with autism learn and understand language, process information, and communicate. These concrete cues are very effective, as many children on the autism spectrum respond well to visual information. It allows them to refer back to the information over time and learn at their own pace.

Communication books or boards are a common example of visual supports that use images and/or words on cards to help the individual learn the word and its meaning. Children can point to the image, helping them communicate their wants or needs. As they learn more symbols and words, they can create sentences and communicate more effectively.

Another example is a visual or picture schedule, which helps individuals learn the steps of a routine or task, like getting ready for bed. The series of pictures shows steps in order, and over time, they learn each step. Visual schedules can also be used to show changes in routine, which helps children on the spectrum prepare for change, cope with it more easily, and understand the language surrounding the change.

About Language

Language is a complex system that enables people to communicate and express ideas through words and their arrangement, whether they are spoken, written, or nonverbal. It facilitates the sharing of knowledge, emotions, and experiences between individuals.

Receptive

When we talk about receptive language, we are referring to how well your child can comprehend and understand language. This could include understanding simple instructions, following conversations, and processing the information that is presented to them.

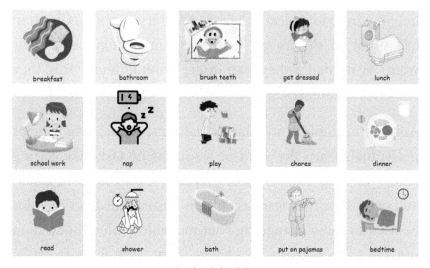

Daily Schedule

Expressive

A child's expressive language is their ability to communicate their thoughts and feelings. This skill allows them to express their needs and wants, share ideas, and connect with others. Expressive language skills can be used to articulate emotions, opinions, and desires with clarity and confidence.

Speech

Speech is a form of communication that involves the use of verbal language. It is the process of conveying thoughts, ideas, and emotions through the production of sounds that are formed into words. These words are then organized and arranged into meaningful sentences to create an effective message.

Nonverbal methods

Non-verbal communication refers to the exchange of information without using spoken or written language. It includes various forms of communication, such as body language, gestures, facial expressions, eye contact, touch, and posture. These non-verbal cues can convey emotions, attitudes, and intentions that words may not be able to express adequately.

Pragmatics

Pragmatics refers to how language is used in various social situations. It encompasses the unwritten rules of communication, such as turn-taking, understanding implicit meanings, and contextually appropriate language use. The ability to accurately interpret and apply pragmatic rules can make a significant difference in how we communicate and connect with others.

Augmentative and Alternative Communication (AAC)

Augmentative and alternative communication (AAC) helps children who have difficulty speaking or are hard to understand. It encompasses all forms of communication besides verbal speech. AAC provides an alternative for individuals to communicate effectively, even if they struggle with speech or language skills. Using AAC can be especially beneficial for autistic children, as well as for developing spoken communication skills. AAC devices can be obtained with the aid of therapists and children's hospitals. Some people may worry that using AAC can hinder speech development or prevent someone from speaking altogether, but research shows that this is not the case (LeafWing Center, 2021). Rather, AAC can actually aid in language development and help individuals improve their reading and writing skills.

Sign Language

Sign language is a communication method that involves hand signals, facial expressions, and body language to express oneself. For individuals with autism who struggle with traditional verbal language or understanding and expressing emotions, sign language can be a highly effective communication tool. American Sign Language (ASL) and British Sign Language (BSL) are examples of different sign languages that have their own unique grammar and vocabulary. Some simplified sign language systems, such as Picture Exchange Communication System (PECS) and Makaton, use pictures or symbols to aid in communication and have been shown to greatly assist children with autism.

Gestures

Gestures are a powerful way for children with autism to communicate when they struggle with words or expressing emotions. Pointing at objects or pictures, thumbs up or down for approval or disapproval, waving for attention, clapping for excitement, or ending an activity, opening and closing hands for "yes" or "no," and touching their chest for comfort or a hug are common gestures that can be helpful for autistic children. Touching their ears can indicate that the child needs a break from sensory stimulation.

Pictures, Photos, Objects, and Videos

Autistic children can benefit from using pictures, photographs, objects, and videos to help them understand and express their needs and interests. These tools can help them learn abstract concepts, such as speed, using real objects like toy cars. Photos of common items, like a glass of water, can help a child understand the concept of thirst. Videos are also helpful in teaching social skills, facial expressions, and emotions, with videos of facial expressions being particularly useful in teaching children to recognize and interpret them.

Written Words

For children with autism who can read or are learning to read, written words can be an effective tool for communication and learning. Visual schedules can be created using written words to outline their daily routine and upcoming activities, providing structure and predictability. Social stories, which are written descriptions of social situations, can guide appropriate behaviors and be customized to address specific struggles. Communication books with written words, pictures, or symbols can aid in expressing needs and preferences. Written instructions, such as a recipe, can also be used to provide guidance for completing tasks.

Computers, Tablets, and Other Devices

Electronic devices, such as computers and tablets, can aid communication for autistic children. Speech-generating devices can help develop speech patterns and visuals, while customized educational apps and games can target specific areas of difficulty. Other electronic tools, like noise-canceling headphones and weighted blankets, can regulate sensory input and help reduce sensory overload.

Guidelines for Nonverbal Autistic Children

Children with autism have the ability to communicate in their own unique way, and it's crucial to encourage social interaction to help them learn language skills. Playing games that your child enjoys can be an enjoyable way to promote social interaction. Singing, reciting nursery rhymes, and gentle roughhousing can also be beneficial. When communicating with your child, get close to them by crouching down so that your voice and face are closer, increasing eye contact opportunities.

Imitating your child's sounds and play behaviors can encourage more interaction and vocalizing and promote turn-taking. However, it's important to only imitate positive behaviors, not negative ones. Focusing on nonverbal communication, like gestures and eye contact, is also essential. Respond to your child's gestures and hand them the toy they are pointing to or playing with.

Allow your child time to talk and express themselves without interrupting. Using short and literal phrases can help them learn and understand new vocabulary. Follow their interests and engage them in conversation about what they are doing. Using assistive technologies and visual supports, such as devices and apps with pictures that your child can touch to produce words, can also aid in language development. Additionally, they can use pictures to express their thoughts and requests to you or others.

COMMUNICATION BARRIERS

ASD has no cure, but treatment can help children on the spectrum learn how to communicate—early intervention makes a significant difference. The process of communicating with autistic children isn't always straightforward, and there are no rules to guarantee success. Nevertheless, healthcare providers and mental health experts have gained valuable insights into how to best connect with children who have ASD. It is possible to break down barriers and allow people to reach their full potential with the right approach.

The 11 Communication and Interaction Tips for ASD

Interacting with a child who has ASD can be challenging, but it can also be rewarding. Here are some communication and interaction tips for ASD from the University of Rochester Medical Center (2019):

1. It is important to be patient because it takes a child with ASD longer to process information. You may need to slow down your conversation to match their speed. Long pauses can also be helpful.
2. Help your child learn how to communicate their anger in a constructive way that is not overly aggressive. It's important for them to understand that it is acceptable to express their frustration rather than bottle it up inside.
3. Sometimes, children with ASD have difficulty showing and controlling their emotions. Be persistent but resilient. They may respond bluntly, so try not to take their words personally.
4. Children who have autism tend to respond better to positive reinforcement. It is important to

acknowledge and reward good behavior frequently to help establish and maintain positive habits.

5. Ignore attention-seeking behavior that might irritate you. It is more beneficial to ultimately prevent it by ignoring it rather than reacting. Also, discuss and reward good behavior as often as you can.

6. Interact with your child through physical activity because they tend to have short attention spans. Running around and playing outside can be more engaging and relaxing.

7. Most autistic children need affection, but some may not like to be touched. Respect their personal space, and never force physical contact on them. Be affectionate yet respectful of their preferences and boundaries.

8. Neurodivergent children can struggle with communicating their emotions, but it's important that they feel your love and support. Make sure to show your affection and take an interest in their lives on a regular basis.

9. Your child possesses exceptional skills and a fresh viewpoint that can show you different approaches to perceiving the world. Take the opportunity to gain knowledge from them.

10. It is okay to take a break and seek support from parent support groups or family and friends. Don't forget to take care of yourself. School psychologists and counselors can also offer helpful resources.

11. It's important to remember that a child with autism is just like any other child, first and foremost. While they may have unique challenges, it's important to believe in their potential and not limit it based on their diagnosis. Keep an open mind and look for opportunities for growth and development.

Listening Skills

Children who are on the autism spectrum often struggle with the ability to focus on the words and meaning of others. They may become distracted by extraneous sounds or more interesting things in the environment around them. Additionally, the individual speaking may have difficulty capturing and maintaining the attention of the autistic child, as they could be competing with the child's inner thoughts. This can be a significant challenge for autistic individuals, as it can impact their ability to form and maintain relationships and fully participate in social interactions.

Here are a few tips for improving listening skills with children who have ASD. First, to make a message more captivating, it can be helpful to make it interactive. This can be achieved by asking the child to physically follow along with the instructions and adding a rhythmic element to the message. Repetition is also important, both in terms of repeating yourself if the child isn't paying attention and having them repeat your words to confirm understanding.

Breaking instructions down into small steps is another effective way to improve communication with neurodivergent children. Taking frequent pauses and ensuring that the child fully comprehends each step before moving on to the next one can help. It can also be helpful to vary the setting in which you practice communication skills, such as by pausing a TV show and asking the child to recall the order of events they just watched.

Another factor to consider is the child's diet. Sometimes, changing their diet to include healthy sensory foods tailored to their preferences, such as crunchy, squishy, runny, or soft foods, can improve listening skills. Finally, it can be helpful to establish a regular exercise routine to help children with excess energy control their impulses and make it easier for them to sit still and listen when needed.

COMMUNICATING WITH A CHILD WHO HAS ASPERGERS

Children with autism spectrum disorder have unique ways of communicating because no two individuals with autism are alike. Some children may use spoken language, while others may be non-verbal and unable to speak. Some children may use noises, facial expressions, or Makaton language. Some may use communication devices or picture exchange communication systems (PECs). Some children may communicate through their behavior. It's important to keep in mind that all forms of communication are meaningful, and you should focus on the methods that work best for the individual to facilitate effective communication. Some of the best approaches for children with Asperger's are a minimal speech approach using short and simple sentences, communication devices and AAC, social stories, and speech and language therapy (SpecialKids.Company, 2021).

Be patient and kind when communicating with a child with Asperger's. They likely require more time to process the information you are sharing with them, and may also experience sensory issues that make communication more challenging. Encourage positive communication by offering praise and positive reinforcement, and consider using other rewards. Additionally, be prepared to be flexible in your approach, as children with Asperger's often struggle with change and adapting to new situations. Finding effective communication methods may require trial and error, so keep an open mind and try different strategies until you find what works best for you and your child.

Danielle's Breakthrough

I am happy to share a heartwarming story about a child with Asperger's and how technology helped them communicate better. This story came to me through networking with fellow caregivers and is a great example of how technology can positively impact the lives of those on the spectrum.

Danielle was having difficulty communicating in traditional ways, often becoming frustrated when she could not express herself as they wanted. She started to hit other children when they were interacting because she was frustrated. The school became a problem, and none of her teachers knew how to handle her. As parents, we stopped participating in social events because of Danielle's meltdowns. We saw many psychiatrists and other specialists, but no one had a diagnosis or a plan to help. Finally, when she was eight, Danielle was diagnosed with Asperger's. We saw her diagnosis as a blessing because it gave us the tools to understand what was happening and the support that we needed. When introduced to a tablet with communication apps, Danielle's world changed dramatically. With the help of these apps, she was finally able to communicate her thoughts and feelings. Her tablet also gave Danielle a greater sense of independence and control over her interactions with others. She no longer had to rely on someone else to interpret her words or gestures, and this really helped boost her confidence and self-esteem.

Overall, this story is a testament to the power of technology to help those with autism live more fulfilling lives. By providing new and innovative tools, we can empower people of all abilities to express themselves and connect with others in ways that were previously impossible. It is also a reminder that a diagnosis is not a bad thing—it can help you see the big picture and give your child the tools they need to succeed.

KEY POINTS AND TAKEAWAYS

This section has delved into the communication strategies for autistic children, which tie into Pillar Two, aiming to enhance their inherent potential and promote character development. It's crucial to keep in mind that each child is unique, and the right approach may involve trying different techniques. Giving praise for effective communication and allowing ample processing time are crucial aspects. It's important to remember that behavior is a form of communication too.

Various methods, such as gestures, visual aids, and assistive technology, can facilitate interaction with your child and help them communicate with others. In the next chapter, we will discuss Pillars One and Three, which together form a comprehensive approach to tackling specific challenges. Although together they form a Five Pillar approach, it's important to note that they are not sequential steps but rather a framework to address specific challenges. Pillar One provides insight into understanding your child with ASD and effectively implementing the strategies outlined in this book. Pillar Three will cover methods to manage your child's behavior, including those related to sensory issues and repetitive or aggressive behavior. We'll begin by discussing why these behaviors may arise and then outline ways to address them collaboratively.

4

HANDLING THEIR OBSESSIVE AND REPETITIVE BEHAVIOR

Don't think that there's a different, better child 'hiding' behind autism. This is your child. Love the child in front of you. Encourage his strengths, celebrate his quirks, and improve his weaknesses, the way you would with any child.

— CLAIRE LAZEBNIK

FROM WHY TO WISE

In this chapter, we will discuss the reasons behind the development of obsessions and repetitive behaviors in children with ASD and how to manage them effectively. This topic relates to both Pillar One and Pillar Three of the Five Pillar framework. Understanding why these behaviors occur is necessary before devising a plan to address them. Repetitive behaviors and obsessions are common in children on the spectrum and can serve as a source of comfort in a world that can be overwhelming to them. These behaviors can also be functional and serve a purpose. However, they can interfere with a child's daily life and cause distress to themselves and others around them. Developing effective strategies to manage these behaviors is possible. Together, we will explore various approaches like behavioral interventions, alternative therapies, and medication. By implementing these strategies, parents and other caregivers can help autistic children thrive and improve their quality of life.

THE PRESENCE OF REPETITIVE BEHAVIORS AND RESTRICTED INTERESTS

People with ASD often develop intense interests that can vary widely, from everyday TV shows to more specialized technical or academic topics like computers, trains, science, or historical events (Durham Region Autism Services, 2023a). These interests may seem unusual, focusing on specific details such as numbers, shapes, or patterns, but they can provide structure, order, and predictability for those with ASD. Additionally, these interests can serve as a foundation for social interaction. It's important to avoid labeling these interests as unhealthy and instead encourage exploration while monitoring for signs of distress or obsessive behavior. Repetitive behaviors like hand-flapping, finger-flicking, rocking, or jumping may seem concerning, but they play a therapeutic role for individuals with ASD who may experience sensory distortions and require this type of stimulation or distraction.

Routines and Resistance

Individuals with autism often struggle with the complexities of the world around them due to difficulties with social interactions and sensory overload. To cope with this, they often rely on fixed routines, specific routes, and rituals to navigate daily life. These routines provide a sense of predictability and structure, which can help manage anxiety and confusion. As a result, individuals with autism tend to develop a strong attachment to routines and sameness.

However, the degree of attachment can vary, and even minor changes can cause significant distress. Therefore, it is essential to inform them of any upcoming changes or provide schedules to help them adjust to disruptions. During times of increased stress, such as the holiday season, their dependence on routines may intensify. While it is important to allow this reliance on routines, it should be monitored to ensure it does not become unhealthy, akin to obsessive behavior.

Obsessions

Children and teenagers with ASD tend to have more intense and focused interests than neurotypical children. These interests may include collecting stamps or balls, wanting to know the birthday of everyone they meet, or repeatedly opening and closing doors (Families for Life, 2021). Older children may have narrow interests in a specific topic, like trains, and want to learn everything about it. Some children change interests frequently, while others may maintain the same interest from early childhood through adolescence and into adulthood.

Rituals

Certain neurodivergent children may engage in ritualistic behaviors. For instance, your child may store a cherished object in a specific location, such as the left-hand corner of a shelf in their bedroom. They may need to take it out and touch it before going to bed. Alternatively, they may limit themselves to eating from a particular plate or ask the same questions and always require a specific response.

Routines

Children with autism often rely on routines. They may prefer to eat, sleep, or leave the house using a specific sequence every time (Families for Life, 2021). A consistent bedtime routine, for example, may help your child sleep better. Altering the routine can cause difficulty settling in some cases. Some children may become upset if their regular route home is changed or if they have to deviate from a particular order when dressing each morning.

How Do They Help?

Children with autism spectrum disorder often engage in repetitive behaviors and talk about their specific interests. While this may seem unusual to others, for a child with ASD, it can be a source of enjoyment and comfort. Repetitive behaviors can also provide a way for children with limited play skills to occupy themselves.

Furthermore, routines, rituals, and repetitive behaviors can serve as coping mechanisms that help regulate stress and anxiety. They provide a sense of control over unpredictable surroundings while also offering a way to regulate emotions.

Repetitive behaviors can also serve to regulate sensory input. For instance, children may engage in self-regulatory behaviors like rocking to stimulate their senses and increase sensory input, which helps them relax and feel comfortable (Healis Autism Centre, 2022).

Repetitive behaviors can also be a form of self-expression for children with ASD. For instance, hand flapping can be a way for them to express their excitement or frustration when they may not have the words to do so.

In summary, repetitive behaviors serve several purposes for individuals with autism, and they can be important for emotional and behavioral well-being.

Corrections

For autistic children, repetitive behaviors can be helpful, so trying to completely stop them may not be effective. Instead, finding a balance between acceptance and change may be more effective. However, if the behaviors hinder learning or socialization, intervention may be necessary. Understanding the causes and finding alternative ways to fulfill needs is important. For example, managing sensory issues or finding alternative calming strategies can help. Modeling appropriate play behavior or using behavioral techniques may also be helpful. Encouraging socialization with others who share similar interests can also help.

MANAGING BEHAVIOUR

Understand

For children with autism, obsessions, repetitive behavior, and routines are often significant and meaningful as they help them manage their anxiety and establish some sense of control over a world that can be confusing and chaotic. In some cases, this behavior can assist individuals with sensory issues. To determine the cause of the behavior and its purpose, it is important to closely examine it. For instance, if the person with autism struggles to cope with a specific environment, such as a classroom, it may be because of the lighting. Turning off strip lighting and relying on natural daylight might be a solution.

Modify

To improve independence and reduce potential risks during behavioral episodes, it may be worth considering structural changes to your home or yard. By altering the environment, you can mitigate certain triggers that may cause outbursts. The changes don't have to be extensive, but they should be tailored to your specific situation. Additionally, creating a calm and organized space with designated areas for activities can soothe anxiety and promote relaxation.

Structure

To help a child with ASD cope with change and lessen their reliance on repetitive behaviors, increasing structure is useful. By reducing unstructured situations, like social events, the child can experience less anxiety and feel more comfortable. Gradually loosen routines as the child gets older and adjust them to fit their evolving needs. It's also important to praise the child each time they adapt well to change, which can help build their confidence and encourage positive behavior. With a consistent and supportive approach, children with ASD can learn to navigate changes with more ease and flexibility.

Early Intervention

Repetitive behaviors, obsessions, and routines can be difficult to modify if they persist for a long time. This is why it's crucial to address any problematic behaviors from an early age by setting boundaries and limits, as behaviors that are acceptable in young children may not be appropriate in older children and adults. You should monitor your child's behavior as they grow older and be on the lookout for any new behaviors that may emerge. By setting limits early, you can help your child develop healthy behaviors that will serve them well throughout their life.

Boundaries

When necessary, establish clear and consistent boundaries, such as limiting access to an object, setting a time limit for discussing a topic, or restricting certain behaviors to specific locations. To promote successful behavioral change while minimizing distress, it is best to begin with small, gradual steps, increasing time limits and introducing more restrictions slowly over time.

Collaborate with your child to establish a realistic goal and develop a plan for achieving that goal over a set period of time. Focusing on small, attainable objectives can help build confidence and reinforce success (National Autistic Society, 2020a).

Analyze the root cause of the behavior in question. It may be necessary to work on reducing the amount of time spent on it if the child is unable to stop the behavior entirely. If the issue is that they continue to engage in the behavior throughout the day, even when trying to focus on other tasks, it may be necessary to work on decreasing the frequency. If the problem is a combination of both, start by addressing one aspect to increase the chances of success while minimizing anxiety.

Example

Week 1: Set the plan and goal together and create visual support to explain the behavioral change.

Week 2: The child is allowed to talk about their favorite topic for 20 minutes every hour.

Week 3: The child is allowed to talk about their favorite topic for 15 minutes every hour.

Week 4: The child is allowed to talk about her favorite TV program for 15 minutes every two hours.

Alternatives

Consider suggesting different activities for the person to engage in if they have already talked to their family about their interests for the day. This could include recording their thoughts on their phone or writing them down in a notebook. Even if the family is not participating, their thoughts are still being expressed, which may help alleviate their anxiety. You can use visual aids to explain these different options.

It may also be worthwhile to explore new ways for the person to engage with their interests, such as by joining a club or group, or pursuing related studies or work. If the interest relates to sensory needs, offer alternative activities that serve the same purpose.

Repeated Verbal Phrases

Children, teenagers, and adults may repeat phrases for various reasons. These reasons could include wanting to reduce anxiety or seeking attention. It's essential to understand that sometimes these reasons can overlap. To address this behavior, strategies such as implementing visual schedules to reduce anxiety or interrupting and redirecting with structured questions can be helpful (Watson Institute, 2023).

Visual Schedules

A visual schedule that uses pictures, words, or objects to sequence events or activities provides a sense of structure and routine, which can be particularly helpful for autistic children with certain behavioral challenges, such as repeated verbal phrases. They can better anticipate what will happen next and when activities will end—this can prevent stress and anxiety, and reduce the likelihood of challenging behaviors. Using a visual schedule can also promote independence, improve communication, and foster positive interactions between children, their caretakers, and their environments.

Interrupting and Redirecting

To guide a child away from stereotypical behaviors, interruption, and redirection techniques can be used. Instead of physically or verbally blocking the child, a structured verbal choice question can be asked, such as "Would you like _____ or _____?" (Watson Institute, 2023). This approach provides a sense of control to the child and offers alternative options, preventing or redirecting problematic behaviors. Attention is given only when appropriate replacement behaviors are exhibited, rather than during repetitive behavior. This method is effective in preventing or de-escalating disruptive behaviors.

RESPONDING TO OTHERS

Parents of children with autism often find themselves in uncomfortable situations when encountering strangers. Despite increased awareness about autism, strangers can still be insensitive, rude, or misinformed. This can be even more stressful for parents of children with autism who feel a strong need to defend and protect their child. These encounters with strangers can be confusing and harmful for both parents and children, causing psychological distress (Ryan, 2010). Since it's not immediately obvious whether a child is misbehaving or displaying autism-related behaviors, negative comments towards children with autism are common due to public misunderstanding about autism symptoms (Gray, 2002).

The 5 W's

Assess the situation before deciding how to respond to a stranger who makes a rude or inappropriate comment. One useful approach from Stages Learning is to use the "Five Ws" method and answer five questions about the situation: What, Who, Where, When, and Why (2022). You can better decide how to respond by identifying the core of the comment and who is speaking. The person may have had personal experience with autism that has influenced their attitude, or they could be simply ignorant about it. Try to remain calm and rational, and decide if it's best to ignore their rude comment or take the opportunity to educate and inform the person. You ultimately want to act in the best interest of your child.

What

First, assess exactly what action or behavior is being communicated to you by the stranger. When children are publicly stigmatized, parents are often hurt by actions such as staring, whispering, or being directly asked about their child in a disapproving tone (Gray, 2013). Social avoidance, inappropriate staring, and rude comments are the most frequent behaviors mentioned as hurtful (Gray, 2002). Try to identify and acknowledge the specific behavior being displayed by the other person.

Who

Take a moment to assess the person you are talking to. Determine whether they are an adult or a child and if they are open to revising their views and listening to your response. Consider their emotional state and how it may influence their behavior. Use your judgment to be thoughtful and poised while prioritizing your child's needs. Understanding your conversational partner better will lead to more successful interactions.

When

Are you rushing to an appointment or taking a stroll on a weekend afternoon? It's important to consider your priorities at the moment. Is it the right time to engage with the stranger and address their comments? These are factors to weigh before deciding on your response.

Where

Take note of your physical surroundings in the situation that is unfolding. Are you on a crowded bus or on the beach by the ocean? Observe who is nearby, such as a supportive network of familiar faces or unfriendly strangers. Consider if there are other parents nearby or if you have witnesses to the encounter. Determine if the person you are confronting is still facing you or if you can bring them back for an intelligent conversation.

Why

Consider the person's motivations and intentions. Why are they saying or doing what they are? Are they being rude or ignorant intentionally? Are they making an accusation or feeling entitled to information? You'll want to attempt to understand their underlying beliefs and biases—this can help you better navigate the conversation and find common ground.

The person you are speaking to may have never met someone with autism and may be unaware of how their words can impact others. Or, they might feel entitled to comment on your child's behavior without regard for your feelings. They could come from a country where people with autism are treated differently, or they may have personal experiences that have influenced their opinions in unacceptable ways.

By understanding their motivations and viewpoints, you can better navigate the conversation and respond with empathy and education. It's important to stand up for your child and educate others about autism while also maintaining respect for others.

WISE

One tool that can be used to handle insensitive remarks is "W.I.S.E. Up!", originally created for adopted children and their families. It teaches parents and children how to respond to uncomfortable inquiries and insensitive responses by using four approaches: Walk away, ignore, or change the subject, share what you are comfortable sharing, and educate (Singer, 2010). In some situations, you can choose to share information about your child's autism and behaviors, or use it as an opportunity to educate the person making the remark. Walking away or ignoring the comment are also options. As an ambassador, you can take control of the dialogue and potentially influence the person's beliefs.

Background Research

Gray's research (2002) indicates that parents of children with autism often perceive societal views of their children as unintelligent, undisciplined, and rude. Additional studies have highlighted the difficulties families face when taking their autistic child to public places and how they use emotional regulation to conceal their discomfort (Ryan, 2010). In a study by Broady, Stoyles, and Morse (2015), four areas of stigmatizing experiences for families with autistic children were identified: lack of knowledge, judgment, rejection, and lack of support. These experiences were found in various contexts, and individuals who experienced stigma in one setting often faced it in others. Therefore, more support is necessary to assist parents in developing effective strategies to cope with discrimination in different situations.

KEY POINTS AND TAKEAWAYS

This chapter focused on managing the behavior of autistic children by understanding the reasons behind their repetitive and obsessive traits. Obsessions and routines provide order and can regulate sensory input, making them beneficial to the child. It is important to find a balance between accepting and modifying these behaviors.

Once you have a good understanding of why your child acts in a particular way, you can collaboratively develop strategies to manage their obsessions and routines. These measures may include interventions, adjustments, or alternatives. The chapter also outlines how to deal with strangers who stigmatize your child due to their behavior. Depending on the situation, you can opt to educate and address their response or ignore it and walk away instead.

This chapter is closely linked to Pillars One and Three of the Five Pillar framework, as its content covers the reasons behind your child's behavior (Pillar One) and ways to manage it (Pillar Three). While this chapter has discussed obsessions and routines, the next one will explore aggressive behavior in depth, which is also connected with Pillars One and Three.

Let's Take A Breath...

"Sometimes, all a parent needs to know [is that] the impossible is actually possible. Hope goes a long way when it comes to autism."

— *LIZ BECKER*

You're taking in a lot of information here, so let's take a breather to remember that you're not alone.

As we discussed in the introduction, ASD is often hidden, and we aren't always aware of the number of people it affects. The same is true of parents – it's easy to think we're part of a very small group of people raising children with autism... But the World Health Organization estimates that one in every hundred children has it.

Even if you know other parents in a similar boat, it's easy to feel isolated, and like other parents don't understand the struggles you're going through... but there are more people out there like you than you probably realize... and you're in a unique position to show them that they're not alone.

By leaving a review of this book on Amazon, you'll show other parents where they can find the guidance they're looking for – and let them know they're not alone in the process.

Simply by letting other readers know how this book has helped you and what they'll find inside, you'll point them in the direction of the support they're looking for, and you'll remind them that there are other parents in exactly the same boat.

Thank you so much for your support. I know you understand how isolating this journey can feel, and I'm grateful to you for joining me in my mission to provide this support to as many parents as I can.

Scan the QR code to leave review!

5

MANAGING AGGRESSIVE BEHAVIOR

Kids who are oppositional or acting out in angry and aggressive ways often can't explain how they're feeling. They are overwhelmed, yet the only emotion they know how to communicate is anger.

— TRICIA GOYER

THE FIRST STEP IS UNDERSTANDING

Children with autism not only struggle with social communication difficulties, restricted interests, and sensory processing issues but also display other autism-related behaviors, such as aggression.

Aggressive behavior in autism can take various forms, like severe tantrums, anger, hostility, self-harm, and destructive behavior, affecting the daily functioning and quality of life of individuals with autism and their caregivers. Up to 20% of individuals with autism display such violent behaviors (Thinking Autism, 2021). This chapter aims to provide parents and caregivers of children with autism with insights into the causes of aggressive behavior and effective strategies to manage it, drawing from Pillars One and Three of the Five Pillar framework. Pillar One helps caregivers understand the underlying causes of their ASD child's behavior, while Pillar Three provides practical strategies for managing their child's behavior, including positive reinforcement, visual aids, and sensory interventions. The chapter explores the underlying reasons for aggressive behavior in children with autism, and the strategies aim to prevent aggressive outbursts, de-escalate intense situations, and promote positive behaviors in their children, empowering caregivers to help their children with autism thrive and live fulfilling lives.

UNDERSTANDING AGGRESSION

Low glucose levels have been linked to aggressive behavior in individuals with autism, as the brain areas responsible for managing negative behavior rely heavily on glucose (Gailliot & Baumeister, 2007). Self-control requires significant energy, much of which comes from glucose, and insufficient levels can lead to reduced self-control and impulsive behavior (Thinking Autism, 2021). Other factors contributing to aggressive behavior in autism include physical pain, sensory disruptions, and social rejection. To manage aggressive behavior, caregivers must address the underlying causes, including the possible role of low glucose levels.

Risk Factors

Kanne and Mazurek's (2010) study examined whether the same risk factors for aggression in neurotypical children apply to those with autism. The study found that male gender, lower parental education, lower IQ, and lower language or communication ability were not associated with the risk of aggressive behavior in autistic children. Instead, younger age, severe social difficulties, repetitive behaviors (such as self-injurious or ritualistic behaviors or resistance to change), and average family income were associated with aggression in children with ASD (Anderson, 2015). Higher family income was surprisingly linked to a higher risk of aggression, potentially because of better access to challenging interventions that can lead to aggressive behavior or a difference in reporting behavior based on income levels.

Functions of Aggression

Before trying to initiate behavior change, understand the underlying reasons for your child's behavior. This can have a positive impact on the child and help manage their behavior more effectively. One way to explore the root cause of a child's behavior is to identify the four functions of behavior, as outlined by Behavioral Innovations (2022).

Escape

The child is displaying behavior aimed at escaping or avoiding a task. For example, throwing a tantrum when a caregiver tries to comb their hair.

Attention

The child is behaving in a manner intended to attract the attention of another person, even if it results in negative feedback.

Access

The child is displaying behavior aimed at obtaining physical access to something they desire, such as a toy or video game.

Automatic Reinforcement

The behaviors displayed due to automatic reinforcement are related to things that either provide the child with a sense of pleasure or assist them in regulating their sensory input.

RULES AND DISCIPLINE

Children with autism find comfort in structured routines, making the concept of boundaries crucial for them (Morin, 2022). Establishing rules and limits can reinforce these routines and greatly benefit your child. Children with ASD have unique ways of processing information and interacting with the world, and clear boundaries can provide them with a sense of structure and predictability, promoting feelings of security and confidence. Additionally, boundaries help children with ASD understand their expectations and limitations, reducing their anxiety levels. When faced with unexpected situations, established rules and limits prepare them by providing structure, predictability, and a sense of safety, enabling them to navigate challenges and feel more comfortable in social situations.

Managing Aggressive Behavior

Be Proactive

Parents can take proactive measures to prevent aggressive behavior in their children, which can be highly beneficial. According to Behavioral Innovations (2021), ensuring that children get enough rest is crucial, especially for those who tend to act aggressively when tired. Parents can also establish clear rules regarding access to preferred items, such as electronic devices, to help prevent aggression. For children with sensory processing difficulties, parents can seek alternative ways to satisfy their child's sensory needs without resorting to harmful behaviors. Quality time spent with children is also vital, and parents should set aside time to engage in enjoyable activities with their children. Lastly, parents can assist their children in replacing aggressive behavior with functional communication skills and alternative behaviors. These strategies can help foster a more peaceful and harmonious home environment while reducing the likelihood of aggressive behavior in children.

Reinforcement: Inappropriate Behavior

Avoid unintentionally reinforcing aggressive behavior, as it can increase the likelihood of it happening again in the future. To understand what might be reinforcing the behavior, identify its function. For example, if a child is acting aggressively to obtain a device, giving it to them may reinforce the behavior (Behavioral Innovations, 2022). Caregivers should reflect on their actions to determine if they may be reinforcing aggressive behavior unintentionally. Being mindful of the consequences of one's actions can help reduce the likelihood of aggression and promote a more positive home environment.

Reinforcement: Appropriate Behavior

To guide your child's behavior towards positive conduct, focus on reinforcing desired behavior rather than punishing aggression. Identify alternative behaviors you'd like to see and reinforce them by praising your child for displaying them. This helps establish positive behavior and encourages them to repeat it in the future, creating a safe and positive environment for their development. (Behavioral Innovations, 2022)

Safety

If your child's aggression poses a safety threat, take immediate action. For less severe cases, have a plan in place, set boundaries, and reinforce positive behavior. Address the underlying causes of aggression with counseling or therapy.

Self-Care

Caregiving can be draining, especially when dealing with a child with challenging behavior. Prioritize your well-being by finding a support system of trusted individuals who understand and can provide practical and emotional support. Plan for breaks to recharge, like regular alone time or date nights. It's essential to have others who can help care for your child, like family or babysitters. Remember, taking care of yourself is vital for both your and your child's well-being, as it equips you to handle the demands of parenting.

Rules

Rules set expectations for children and create a positive environment. Use positive statements that focus on what your child can do instead of what they can't. Visual supports are an effective tool, such as using a timer to show when playtime can begin (Raising Children Network Australia, 2020b). Be consistent with enforcing rules and consequences, and provide positive reinforcement for good behavior.

Triggers

Consider keeping a record of your child's behavior after an aggressive incident, including what happened before the behavior, warning signs, specific actions taken, and how you and others responded. Tracking patterns can prevent future incidents and provide valuable information for assessments. Documenting specifics can help parents and caregivers better understand behavior and find effective ways to address it.

Professionals

A behavior analyst can conduct a Functional Behavior Assessment and create a Behavior Support Plan to address your child's problem behaviors. However, these suggestions are not a substitute for professional evaluation and guidance. Seek help from a professional to help your child overcome their frustrations and impulses.

Discipline at School

Collaborating with your child's school to establish a shared approach to discipline has several benefits. When both environments have similar expectations and strategies, children are more likely to understand appropriate behaviors. Working with the school can also provide insights into your child's behavior and facilitate open communication between you and the teachers. This allows for a more coordinated effort to address any issues and support your child's overall well-being (Morin, 2022).

About Time-Out

Time-outs can be effective, but they're not suitable for every child or situation. Parents may make mistakes when using time-outs, such as not following through with the consequence, talking to the child during the time-out, or using an entertaining space (Lee, 2022). To improve their effectiveness, parents should remain calm, avoid anger or yelling, be consistent, and use a quiet space. After the time-out, caregivers should reassure the child and discuss their behavior, explaining why it was inappropriate and how to avoid it in the future. Time-outs should be used appropriately and in combination with positive reinforcement for good behavior.

Alternatives

Parents and caregivers should balance demands and reinforcement and prioritize positive reinforcement over time-outs when managing problematic behavior. Dr. Mary Barbera suggests creating eight positive experiences for every negative consequence (2022). This involves praising good behavior, offering rewards for tasks, and creating a supportive environment. Parents can promote good behavior by setting clear boundaries, providing consistent positive reinforcement, and identifying underlying issues. Positive reinforcement does not mean ignoring negative behavior but addressing it constructively. For further useful information, you can follow Dr. Barbera on Facebook at MaryBarbera.com/facebook.

IF THEY HIT YOU

Neutral redirection is an ABA technique that replaces aggressive behavior with appropriate actions in autistic children (Therapeutic Pathways, 2021). By using this approach, parents can help their children learn socially acceptable behavior and improve their interactions with peers. To use neutral redirection, remain calm, avoid reacting, and redirect your child to a different method of communication. Refrain from giving attention to aggressive behavior and prepare other children on how to respond to their sibling's aggressiveness.

Understanding

Aggressive behavior in autistic children can be caused by a range of factors, including sensory overload or difficulty communicating their feelings. Parents can help by monitoring their child's emotions and encouraging the use of learned communication techniques. Seeking help from a licensed behavioral therapist is recommended for children who engage in aggressive behavior. It's important to stick with new behavior strategies, as these behaviors may worsen before improving. By teaching children that hitting no longer achieves their desired outcome, the negative behavior will lose its function and lead to positive changes.

Yelling

Yelling at children with autism is ineffective and can increase their stress levels, which can exacerbate their behavior and aggression challenges. Instead, families can work with behavioral interventionists to learn effective strategies for managing behavioral challenges at home. Children with autism naturally experience higher levels of stress and struggle with situational awareness, impulse control, and understanding social norms. Yelling can lead to depression and negatively impact their emotional well-being (Tatom, 2022).

How to Stop

Aggressive behavior in autistic children can create challenges for caregivers and have negative long-term consequences. Understanding the reasons behind the behavior and seeking professional help can lead to identifying sensory needs and positive coping strategies. ABA therapy can take several years to master, and seeking support from other professionals is essential (Tatom, 2022).

DEVELOPING PATIENCE

Raising a child with autism requires patience, and planning and preparation can alleviate chaos and frustration. The Autism Site suggests remaining calm during repetitive behaviors, seeking support, doing something relaxing, empathizing with your child's perspective, breaking down hurdles into smaller steps, focusing on positive behaviors, seeking refuge, and considering respite care (2017). Coping techniques, planned responses, and support resources can help cultivate patience and help you become the best caregiver for your child with autism.

BRETT & TIFFANY'S SHIFT

Tiffany's son Brett was a good student and spoke fluently, but when he got angry, he would lash out at his family members, throw things, and even bang his head against the wall. This was a source of constant stress and worry, especially because Brett shared a bedroom with his younger brother. Tiffany had to separate the boys on several occasions because she was afraid Brett would hurt his brother during one of his outbursts.

But it wasn't just his aggression that concerned Tiffany. Brett had a sleep disorder that caused him to wake up frequently during the night, which only made his behavior worse. Tiffany tried everything she could think of to help Brett get a better night's sleep. She established a bedtime routine, made sure he had a comfortable and calming environment, and even tried giving him natural sleep aids. But nothing seemed to work.

While doing some research, Tiffany read about a therapy called ABA that involved teaching children with autism how to manage their repetitive behaviors, which could reduce their risk of aggression. She found a local therapist who specialized in this approach and began taking Brett to regular sessions.

Over time, Brett and Tiffany learned how to recognize his triggers and redirect his behavior before he became aggressive. He learned coping strategies like deep breathing and counting to ten. And he learned how to manage his repetitive behaviors, which helped reduce his anxiety and frustration. It wasn't an easy journey, but Tiffany is proud of how far Brett has come. There will be more challenges ahead, but she feels better equipped to handle them now that Brett is getting the help he needs.

KEY POINTS AND TAKEAWAYS

The key concept in this chapter is understanding your child's aggressive behavior, which is often an expression of frustration and overwhelm due to difficulty with communication. Consistent rules and boundaries can reduce anxiety levels and help children with ASD understand their expectations and limitations. Proactively identifying triggers and reinforcing positive behaviors are also effective strategies.

It's important to manage caregiver stress and seek professional support, including therapy. Implementing behavior strategies may take time and initially worsen aggressive behavior. The next chapter will continue to focus on Pillars One and Three, addressing sleep and sensory issues in autistic children. Sleep is crucial for development and well-being, and sensory issues can cause overload and avoidance behaviors. The chapter will explore reasons for sleep difficulties and various sensory challenges, offering practical strategies for better sleep and improved quality of life.

6

DEALING WITH THEIR SENSORY ISSUES AND SLEEP PROBLEMS

There is hope and strength in understanding.

— TEMPLE GRANDIN

SENSES AND SLEEP

Getting enough quality sleep can be a challenge for autistic children, as they may struggle with both falling asleep and staying asleep. Factors such as bedtime routines, sleep, and lifestyle habits can contribute to these issues. In this chapter, we will explore potential solutions to improve the child's sleep quality by making changes to their sleeping environment, routines, and habits.

Addressing sensory processing issues is also crucial, as these sensitivities can greatly impact the child's comfort and well-being. By creating a sensory-friendly bedroom with appropriate lighting, flooring, and calming scents and colors, caregivers can help reduce potential triggers and promote a better sleep environment for the child. Taking an individualized approach to managing sleep and sensory issues is key to promoting a healthier and happier lifestyle for both the child and the family. These strategies correspond to Pillars One and Three of the Five Pillar framework, which aims to help caregivers understand and mitigate their child's behavior.

SENSORY OVERLOAD

Sensory symptoms refer to the way someone behaves in response to their sensory surroundings. As defined by the Carmen B. Pingree Autism Center of Learning, when the amount of input received from one's senses is more than their brain can handle, it is called sensory overload (2021).

Not all children with ASD experience sensory challenges, but many do. Some neurodivergent children experience differences in the way they perceive sensory input from their environment, while others may struggle more intensively with certain sensory experiences. It's important to remember that we all have our own sensory preferences and sensitivities. Different people may respond in contrasting ways to various sensory inputs: You might enjoy the feeling of soft blankets, but someone else may find them uncomfortable (Behavioral Innovations, 2021). Everyone has unique sensory needs and ways of processing sensory information.

Pain

Children with ASD may have a different perception of pain when compared to others. They may not feel pain as intensely as neurotypical individuals do, or they may bear more. For example, some children on the spectrum may not notice a bleeding cut, while others might experience pain more intensely than their peers in the same situation.

Hearing

Autistic children may display an extreme sensitivity to certain sounds that may not bother neurotypical individuals. This heightened sensitivity can cause the child significant distress, leading to anxiety and agitation. While it is normal for all people to dislike certain sounds to some degree, those on the spectrum can experience a much stronger aversion.

Touch

Sensory challenges make certain textures uncomfortable for autistic children. This sensitivity can extend to clothes or objects that they are in contact with, prompting them to avoid such items altogether. This feeling of discomfort can be intense and beyond their ability to cope, making it challenging for them to engage in activities that involve exposure to such textures. Hypersensitivity to certain textures is not unusual among kids or adults with ASD, indicating the need for more specialized support to help them navigate the sensory world effectively.

Smell

Children with ASD may have a particular liking for or dislike for certain smells. Some may find certain smells extremely unpleasant, while others may have an overactive sense of smell that can make life challenging due to being constantly bombarded with smells that bother them. It is important to consider ruling out any medical cause if your child seems to be bothered by certain smells, as this may or may not be related to an allergy (Behavioral Innovations, 2021).

Sight

It is important to pay attention to how your child responds to visual stimulation, as some children may become over-stimulated or distressed by certain visual cues. Children will have different responses to visual stimuli—one might find something enjoyable, while another finds it bothersome. Keep an eye out for any signs of discomfort, and try to adjust the stimulation accordingly.

Sensitivity Differences

Neurodivergent children can experience a variety of sensory symptoms that affect their behavior and daily functioning. These symptoms can be classified as hyper-responsiveness, where a child is overly sensitive to input, or hypo-responsiveness, where a child is under-sensitive to input. Understanding these behaviors can help caregivers provide the most appropriate support and accommodations.

Hypersensitivity

Sensory hypersensitivity is a condition in which an individual experiences exaggerated and intense reactions to their sensory environment. For instance, a child may feel the need to cover their ears when there is even moderate noise in the environment. Such individuals may be over-responsive to certain stimuli, such as sounds, textures, or visual or olfactory stimuli, which can be overwhelming and cause discomfort or distress. This can result in avoidance behaviors or disruptions in daily activities.

Hyposensitivity

Hypoarousal refers to the tendency to exhibit behaviors that are under-responsive to immediate surroundings. Your child may not react appropriately to loud noises or other external stimuli and appear unresponsive, emotionally flat, or even detached from their surroundings.

RELATIONSHIP BETWEEN AUTISM AND SENSORY SENSITIVITY

We know that autism has both genetic and environmental components. A study published by Taylor et al. (2018) in the Journal of the American Academy of Child & Adolescent

Psychiatry, found that the underlying genetics of autism overlap with those that influence abnormal sensory responses. This research provides further evidence that sensory sensitivities are a core feature of autism. The study found that around 85% of the overlap can be attributed to genetic variables, supporting the idea that these sensitivities run in families. Previous research has also shown that parents and siblings of autistic individuals often exhibit milder versions of their sensitivities—the study also found that almost all mothers of children with autism display unusual responses to sensory stimuli, such as light, touch, and sound (Uljarević et al., 2014). While the link between sensory sensitivities and autism is still in the early stages of investigation, these findings highlight the importance of recognizing and addressing sensory processing difficulties in individuals on the spectrum.

Accommodating for Hypersensitivities

Some simple measures can be taken to accommodate hyper-sensitive needs. Dimming the lights can be helpful, as bright lights can be overstimulating. Incandescent lighting can be used instead of fluorescent, as the flickering of fluorescent bulbs can be bothersome to some people. In noisy environments, earplugs or headphones can be provided to help reduce the noise level. Strongly scented products like air fresheners and perfumes can be eliminated as they may cause discomfort for some individuals. It's important to consider personal sensitivities when providing food and clothing options. This means being mindful of the temperature, texture, and fabric materials. Finally, always ask for permission before touching, especially when giving a hug to a child, as some may not like physical contact.

Accommodating Hyposensitivities

There are several ways to support children who struggle with hyposensitivities. One way is by providing visual aids to help them process spoken information and directions—this can be particularly helpful for children who may struggle with verbal instructions. Another way to help is by offering stronger-tasting or textured foods, which can be a great way to provide a variety of sensory experiences while also helping to build a tolerance to different tastes and textures. Sensory-stimulating toys, such as fidgets, can also be useful tools to help children regulate their emotions and focus their attention. Providing opportunities to participate in stimulating activities can also be helpful, as this can help children explore different sensory experiences in a safe and controlled environment. Finally, using a weighted blanket can provide a sense of comfort and security for children who may struggle with sensory processing issues.

SLEEP PROBLEMS

Sleep problems are common among all children, but autistic children, in particular, may have difficulty falling asleep. They may experience issues such as irregular sleeping patterns, staying awake late at night, or waking up very early. Children with ASD may also sleep much less than expected for their age, or be awake for prolonged periods during the night. Additionally, children on the spectrum sometimes get up and engage in activities or make noise for several hours during the night. These sleep difficulties can be challenging for both the child and their caregivers, but there are strategies available to help improve sleep hygiene and the overall quality of rest for neurodivergent children.

The reasons for sleep problems in children with ASD can vary, and can be related to habits before bedtime or during the day. Anxiety, bedwetting, and biological factors can also contribute to sleep difficulties. Additionally, illnesses or health conditions, night terrors and nightmares, restless sleep, snoring, and social communication difficulties can all affect the quality and duration of sleep for autistic children. These challenges can be particularly difficult for parents and caregivers, as sleep deprivation can make managing daily routines and other symptoms of autism more difficult. However, evidence-based strategies can help improve sleep hygiene and overall well-being.

Bedtime Habits

The bedtime routine and sleep environment can play a significant role in children's ability to fall asleep and stay asleep throughout the night. For example, if there is a lot of noise, activity, or excitement before bedtime, it can be harder for children to feel calm and relaxed enough to drift off to sleep. Similarly, if children do things differently each night before bed, they may not get consistent cues that it's time for bed and sleep. Additionally, if they are used to falling asleep somewhere other than their own bed, such as in the family room, they may struggle to fall asleep in their own bed. For children with specific bedtime preferences, such as needing all of their toy cars lined up on the bed before they can sleep, this can create additional challenges if something is missing or out of place. Environmental factors, such as temperature, light, and noise, can also make it difficult to get to sleep, particularly for autistic children who may have sensory sensitivities. By addressing these factors and creating a consistent and calming bedtime routine and sleep environment, parents and caregivers can help children develop healthy sleep habits.

Daytime Habits

Unhealthy eating habits and a lack of physical activity during the day can sometimes contribute to children's sleep problems. Fortunately, simple lifestyle changes can help address these issues. Encouraging them to engage in more physical activity throughout the day, including at least an hour of energetic play like running and jumping, can help promote better sleep. Additionally, ensuring that your child has their evening meal at a time that allows them to go to bed feeling neither too hungry nor too full can also be helpful. It's important to avoid caffeine and excitement in the evening, as well as long and late daytime naps for children over the age of five. By making these lifestyle changes, parents and care-givers can support healthy sleep habits and improve the quality and duration of their children's sleep.

Anxiety

Autistic children who struggle with anxiety may find it hard to fall asleep at night. It's best to avoid discussing any topics that may trigger worries or stress before bedtime to help them get a good night's rest. Instead, try to have conversations with your child about their fears and concerns during the day, when they are better able to process this information. By listening to your child and providing them with opportunities to express themselves, you can help reduce their anxiety and encourage better sleep habits. Creating a calm and soothing bedtime routine can also be helpful in promoting relaxation and preparing your child for a restful night's sleep.

Bedwetting

It is common for children with ASD to experience late toilet training or struggle with toilet training altogether. Bedwetting can also be a problem for these children, causing them to wake up during the night because they are wet. Sizes for Goodnites Underwear are available for individuals weighing up to 140 lbs. Alternatively, they may wake up to use the restroom but then have difficulty falling back asleep. If this is the case for your child, it might be helpful to seek assistance. A good starting point is to speak with your child's therapists. If the problem persists, a visit to your child's doctor may also be necessary.

Biological Causes

For neurodivergent children, sleep problems can also have biological causes. For example, sometimes the hormones in the brain that control sleep are released differently from the way they're released in neurotypical children—this can mean that some autistic children aren't 'tuned in' to their own need for sleep. Speak to your child's doctor if you think this could be affecting your child's sleep.

Illness and Health Conditions

Autistic children, just like all children, can face illnesses such as colds or ear infections, which can disrupt their sleep routine. When a child is sick, their bedtime routine may need to be adjusted. However, once the child is feeling better, it's important to gradually return to the usual bedtime routine. Positive reinforcement can help make this transition smoother.

For individuals with allergies or sensitive skin who want more restful sleep by regulating body temperature, a washable wool mattress pad is highly recommended because of its hypoallergenic and temperature control properties. If you suspect that your child's sleep issues are due to a medical problem such as asthma or epilepsy, it is again important to speak with your child's doctor for further advice.

Night Terrors and Nightmares

Some sleep behaviors that parents may perceive as problematic are actually quite common in all children. Night terrors, which are sudden and intense episodes of agitation during deep sleep, are typically experienced by children between the ages of 2 and 12 and do not indicate a serious problem—similarly, nightmares, which can wake children up and make it difficult for them to fall back asleep, are normal for children of all ages (Raising Children Network Australia, 2020a). However, if you are concerned about your child's sleep behavior or if their behavior appears severe, you can always speak to their doctor for further guidance and support.

Restless Sleep

Autistic children occasionally experience more restless sleep compared to non-autistic children. This may manifest in body-rocking, head-banging, and head-rolling. Even though it is a common condition, it may also indicate less common sleep disorders. If you're worried or your child does not respond to settling techniques, it is best to seek advice from your child's doctor.

Sometimes, autistic children take medicines that have side effects that hinder their sleep routine. It is recommended to also consult with your child's doctor if this may be a problem for your child.

Snoring

Sometimes, children with ASD may snore while sleeping, just like any other child. However, if you notice that your child's snoring is persistent, it is important to consult your child's doctor. This is because persistent snoring could indicate a condition called sleep apnoea, which may require medical attention.

Social Communication Difficulties

Children with autism may experience sleep problems due to challenges in social communication, which can make it difficult for them to express their needs and wants, ultimately leading to trouble falling or staying asleep. Therefore, it is recommended to work on improving your child's communication skills to help alleviate sleep issues. Additionally, social communication difficulties may hinder your child's ability to recognize bedtime cues from family members. In such cases, establishing a consistent and positive bedtime routine can help your child understand when it's time for sleep.

Impact of Sleep Problems

The quality of sleep that a child receives significantly impacts their health and overall well-being. Inadequate sleep is correlated with behaviors such as aggression, depression, hyperactivity, increased behavioral issues, irritability, and poor cognitive performance in children with autism. It is likely that your sleep is also affected if your child is having trouble sleeping (Watson, 2008).

Getting a Good Night's Sleep—Your Child

Getting children to sleep can be a challenge, especially when they have trouble communicating their feelings and worries to their caregivers. This is often the case for children with ASD, who may experience meltdowns close to bedtime when they are tired and overwhelmed. Research shows that good sleep hygiene plays a significant role in helping autistic children fall asleep more quickly and sleep more soundly. The American Academy of Pediatrics recommends behavioral treatments that focus on establishing a calming bedtime routine and creating a soothing sleep environment (Mattei, 2020). Tips for improving sleep hygiene include taking daytime naps earlier in the afternoon and keeping them relatively short; exercising regularly to help manage excess energy; avoiding stimulants like caffeine and nicotine before bedtime; and creating an appropriate bedtime environment that is dark, cool, and free from stimuli or distractions that could disrupt sleep. Establishing a regular bedtime routine that includes relaxing activities like reading a story and avoiding electronic devices has also been shown to be beneficial for neurodivergent children. Additional strategies for improving sleep hygiene include deep pressure simulation, the use of a weighted blanket, and comforting objects like stuffed animals or blankets.

Designing a Bedroom for a Child With ASD

A well-designed bedroom for children with autism should prioritize functionality, sensory needs, safety, and independence while still maintaining a cute and fun aesthetic. Sensory sensitivity can vary among children with autism, and environmental stimuli can provoke severe and destabilizing reactions. To minimize these negative reactions, a child's bedroom should avoid extraneous noise, bright lights, hard edges, intense colors, and chaotic patterns.

Instead, it should create a safe and comfortable space with soft and familiar objects, a cozy bed, play or learning accommodations, and a calming atmosphere that considers every detail:

- Demarcate spaces: To aid in the focus of children with autism, it's essential to provide them with familiar spaces. Dividing their bedroom into specific zones for sleeping, playing, learning, and leisure can help achieve this. The bed should be away from the window with controlled lighting, while play, study, and leisure areas should be located closer to the window for natural sunlight.
- Control lighting: Choose lighting carefully for children with sensory issues. Avoid white lights and opt for yellow lights instead. Filter natural light and use blackout curtains or shades to darken the room at night. Install dimmer switches for light control and position lights upward to minimize intensity.
- Choose relaxing colors: Choose bedroom colors carefully, as they can impact mood and function. Opt for calming tones like blue, green, purple, and soft

gray, and avoid over-stimulating bright hues like red, orange, and yellow. Skip distracting patterns and choose non-toxic, washable paint if your child licks surfaces. Lastly, avoid blank white walls, as they can confuse the child's perception of their space.

- Pick quiet flooring: In Atypical's first episode, Sam, an autistic boy, loves Antarctica for its quietness (Magical Nest, 2021). As autistic children are sensitive to sounds, the flooring in their room should be chosen carefully. Natural wood absorbs sound and offers a soft, warm surface, while laminate flooring should be avoided as it can be noisy. Alternatively, solid-colored carpeting or tile carpeting are good options that are easy to install and maintain. Checkerboard patterns should be avoided.

- Plan plenty of storage: To make a room suitable for a child with ASD, organize the space well with different types of storage. Under-bed storage drawers can hide things, while clear stackable drawers should be labeled with symbols or words. Keep breakable items or toys that need supervision in a locked closet.

- Choose the right type of bedding: When choosing bed linen for an autistic child, remember that texture can be a stimulant. Soft, high-thread-count cotton sheets that don't create lumps and can be washed at high temperatures are recommended. Weighted sheets can provide comfort, and color choices can follow the same theory as wall colors. A monochromatic color scheme is highly recommended.

- Be careful with electronics: Avoid TVs or laptops in your child's room due to their addictive and stimulating effects. Remove items that produce loud noises or have many wires. Instead, consider using electronics that project calming images or white noise machines for relaxation and better sleep.

- Minimize visual clutter: For a child's room, a minimalist decor style is best to encourage focus. Limit wall art to one frame per wall, choosing natural landscapes or abstract prints with spirals and soft curves. Avoid any art with sharp lines and angles.

- Create a sensory deprivation area: Create a sensory deprivation area in your child's room with a tent or canopy and include soft pillows, a weighted blanket, noise-canceling headphones, and fidget toys. This helps your child calm down and improve self-regulation.

- Think about the scents: Children with autism can be scent-sensitive. Use natural sources for scents like plants, flowers, and fruits. Open the windows for fresh air. Dilute oils if using an oil diffuser. Citrus and mint energize, while lavender and eucalyptus relax.

- Prioritize safety: Prioritize safety when designing your child's room, especially for those with autism. Lock storage units, doors, and windows. Soften corners and cover sockets. Create special safety measures for your child's unique needs, such as a designated climbing area or an interior child lock.

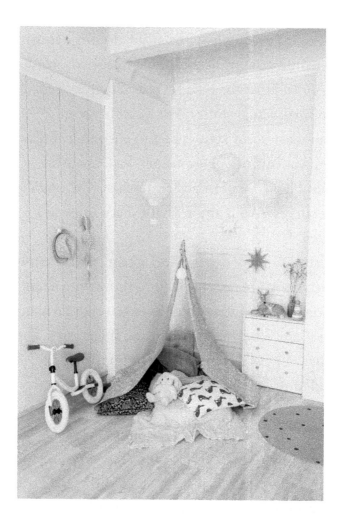

Getting a Good Night's Sleep—You and Your Family

Sometimes it's important to ignore the "shoulds" and "should-nots" you hear about sleep, and focus on what works best for your family in order to help your child get better sleep (National Autistic Society, 2020b). For example, if your child wants to sleep with you, it may be okay to allow it.

Talk to your doctor about medication options, including melatonin. While there isn't long-term evidence for using melatonin, it can be helpful in the short-term to help your child get better sleep (Churchman, 2019). Make sure to discuss this option with your doctor, and consider implementing new routines and practices to eventually wean your child off the medication.

To make sure your child is safe while they sleep, safety-proof their room. Don't feel pressured to sleep when your child sleeps if it's not convenient for you, and don't hesitate to seek help and advice from professionals—especially if you are struggling with a long-term lack of sleep. Getting a good night's sleep is important for both your family and your child, but it can be difficult to achieve.

KEY POINTS AND TAKEAWAYS

Autistic children often struggle with sleep, which can negatively impact their well-being and functioning. It's important to identify and address the factors contributing to their sleep difficulties. Designing a sleep environment that caters to their sensory needs can help mitigate sensory and sleep issues.

In the previous three chapters, we focused on Pillars One and Three, which covered understanding your child's behavior and strategies to help you manage it. Now we will shift our attention back to Pillar Two, which emphasizes the importance of social skills and interactions for children with ASD. Autistic children may struggle to navigate social situations, but with the right support and guidance, they can improve their social skills and form meaningful relationships. We'll provide insights into their unique challenges and needs, as well as effective strategies such as social stories, role-playing, and structured playdates. Building positive relationships and friendships can have a significant impact on their overall well-being and development.

7

HELPING THEM BUILD SOCIAL SKILLS AND FRIENDSHIPS

When a family focuses on ability instead of disability, all things are possible...Love and acceptance is key. We need to interact with those with autism by taking an interest in their interests.

— AMANDA RAE ROSS

FINDING FRIENDSHIP

In this chapter, we will delve into the complex issue of why children with ASD and Asperger's experience difficulties socializing and interacting with others. We will explore the underlying factors that contribute to these challenges and offer effective intervention strategies to help parents and caregivers support children with autism in developing their social skills and making friends.

This chapter corresponds to Pillar Two of the Five Pillar framework, which focuses on character development, discovering potential, and skill improvement. My aim is to equip you and your child with practical tools and techniques that will enable you to help them succeed in their personal and social lives.

We will examine the assimilation and accommodation strategies that can be used to help children with ASD build meaningful relationships and establish long-term friend-ships. These strategies will enable them to navigate social situations confidently, improve their communication skills, and develop their emotional intelligence.

As always, it is crucial to understand that children with ASD and Asperger's have unique challenges—including socially—that require specific approaches. Accordingly, this chapter will provide a comprehensive overview of those challenges, their impact on the social development of your child, and evidence-based interventions that can be implemented to support them.

Overall, this chapter is designed to empower you with the knowledge and skills needed to help your child overcome some of their social difficulties and thrive in their personal and social lives. By implementing the strategies outlined, you will be able to help them build meaningful relationships and establish a strong foundation for long-term success.

ISSUES WITH SOCIAL SKILLS

Children typically learn through imaginative play and incorporate what they observe into their lives, including in social situations where they adjust their behavior to fit in. However, for children with Asperger's and autism, social interactions pose unique challenges. Their brains do not easily register vital interpersonal information, especially subtle cues like body language and tone of voice, resulting in social awkwardness and inappropriate behavior (Durham Region Autism Services, 2023b). Teaching social skills to these children is crucial, but it requires understanding their difficulties. Children on the spectrum struggle with visual processing, abstract reasoning, and emotional regulation, among other issues. By addressing these challenges and providing appropriate support, parents and educators can help children with Asperger's syndrome develop the social skills they need to succeed in social situations.

The Connection Between Social Skills and Autism

ASD is characterized by a combination of traits that can make it extremely difficult for children to acquire basic social skills. Some of these attributes include delays and difficulties in verbal communication, an inability to read non-verbal communication cues, repetitive or obsessive behaviors, and overwhelming sensory inputs (AppliedBehaviorAnalysisEdu.org, 2017). While this deficit is often misread as a desire to avoid people or social situations, most individuals with ASD desperately want to interact with others but simply lack the necessary skills. This frustration can lead to outbursts or inappropriate behavior in social contexts. On the other hand, some individuals with ASD are oblivious to their own communication issues and may inadvertently offend or make others uncomfortable. They may monopolize conversations, stick to specific topics, or shut out external stimuli. It is crucial to understand these challenges and provide appropriate support to help individuals with ASD develop the social skills they need to succeed in social situations.

HELPING YOUR CHILD IN SOCIAL SITUATIONS

Children with Asperger's and autism can be highly effective learners if approached with appropriate strategies. They can use their memory for rules and logical methods to mitigate the challenges they face. To teach skills effectively, several techniques can be employed.

Direct verbal instruction is essential. Neurodivergent children learn best when taught in direct, logical, and linear ways in a structured and academic approach. New strategies should be taught in a clear, concise way with logical steps that can be reviewed often and practiced in a variety of settings to encourage flexibility. A range of skills should also be taught, such as identifying social cues and body language, understanding appropriate social distance and eye contact, and reading the tone of voice (Durham Region Autism Services, 2023b). Children may need help understanding non-literal language, such as metaphors, if needed.

It is essential to reinforce existing problem-solving skills by helping children identify difficult situations and how to apply their learned knowledge. Your child can develop better inference and prediction skills by verbally explaining the cause and effect of their actions. Additionally, emotional coping strategies can assist children in recognizing their feelings and managing anxiety and frustration before they lead to a meltdown. Better self-care techniques, such as practicing good hygiene, may also need to be taught.

Developing a backup plan is important to give children a chance to fall back on an alternative if their initial plans don't work out as expected and to avoid becoming dismayed when results don't happen as predicted. Note that children with autism can struggle to use social skills they have learned in one setting in other situations. To help them use their skills in various settings, practicing social skills in different situations, such as sharing pencils with a friend who visits or sharing pencils with a sibling at a café, can be beneficial (Raising Children Network Australia, 2023).

Enhancing Interactions

Parents and caregivers play a critical role in reinforcing social skills training at home for children with autism. Although therapy sessions and expert interventions can help improve social skills, it is equally important to continue practicing at home to achieve optimal results. Here are some strategies from Kim Barsolo for Autism Parenting Magazine that parents and caregivers can use (2019):

Role-playing is an effective way to help a child learn expected and unexpected behavior in different scenarios. For example, a child can practice going to school before the actual event.

Playing games together with a parent or sibling can also teach a child about the importance of rules, taking turns, and being a good sport. Games like kicking a ball back and forth, Simon Says, Hide and Seek, and simple board games like Jenga or Connect Four are great options.

Watching videos or observing others during social activities, such as going to the dentist, can help a child recognize basic courtesy skills like greeting the doctor and following instructions.

Social stories are another strategy that can help autistic children develop self-care and social skills (Tobik, 2018). These stories illustrate how people behave when interacting with others and the best ways to work with others to solve problems. Social stories can help a child understand the feelings of others, regulate emotions, and cope with unexpected changes. Parents can also learn to write their own social stories based on their child's behavior by familiarizing themselves with the basics of creating social stories, including choosing the types of sentences to be used, creating characters, and identifying the purpose of the story.

By implementing these strategies at home, parents and caregivers can help children with autism spectrum disorders develop and improve their social skills in a safe and supportive environment.

Friends

The future can seem uncertain and overwhelming for parents of children with autism. The question that often weighs heavily on your heart is whether your child will ever be able to make friends. This fear and uncertainty can cause sleepless nights and a host of other concerns, such as whether your child will be able to attend regular school, participate in sports, find a job, and start a family. However, by having realistic expectations and making a game plan, you can help your child build lasting friendships.

One experience demonstrates that with time, patience, and effort, children with autism can indeed develop strong social lives—after overcoming social challenges, their son is now a thriving teenager who attends public high school and enjoys spending time with a small group of friends (Meyers, 2016). While this process was not easy, the rewards of seeing their son enjoy social connections were worth the effort. Parents of autistic children should not give up hope. Your child can develop friendships that will enrich their lives with the right approach and support.

Building Friendships

Building relationships can greatly impact personal growth and well-being, but it can be challenging for individuals with ASD due to difficulties perceiving social cues and responding appropriately. Children with ASD may have few friends and avoid interactions. However, they have many positive qualities to offer others and need opportunities to form meaningful relationships. Employing various strategies can help them build supportive friendships, leading to a happier life and realizing their potential.

Assessing Needs

Differentiating between skill deficits and performance deficits is crucial in determining the appropriate intervention for children's social skills. Sometimes children have skills but do not use them due to various reasons. Adults may mistake skill deficits for performance deficits, blaming the child for lacking motivation. Observing the child's ability to perform a task in multiple settings can help discern between the two. For example, if a child can only initiate conversations with a parent, they may need to learn to apply the skill in other contexts.

Intervention Strategies

To promote positive social interactions for neurodivergent children, accommodation or assimilation strategies, or a combination of both, may be needed depending on the child's needs. Accommodation modifies the environment, like autism awareness training for classmates. Assimilation facilitates skill development. Focusing on one approach without the other can set children up for failure.

Accommodation Strategies

- Offer opportunities related to the child's interests: Encouraging your child to participate in activities aligned with their interests can help them meet like-minded peers and build strong friendships. These activities can provide opportunities to engage in enjoyable activities, showcase skills, and start conversations with others.
- Promote autism awareness: To improve social interactions for children with ASD, educating peers and adults on their needs is helpful. For instance, explaining that some children with autism may not want their belongings touched can prevent misunderstandings. Your child is not being rude by exhibiting different behaviors; they are simply expressing themselves in their own way.
- Find a peer partner: Finding a peer partner for your child in various settings can promote interactions

with other children. Peer partners can help them adapt to new routines and encourage supportive social behaviors.

Assimilation Strategies

- Help them understand what a friend is: To help your child understand good friendships, find common ground, and explain the difference between positive and negative relationships. Keep it simple by saying, "Friends are kind; they ask about your interests and help you when you struggle." Or try asking questions like, "Do you like being with nice people or name-callers?" (Chen, 2022). Give your child plenty of chances to interact and teach them social skills. Depending on their needs, it may be best to start with a few friendships before exploring the theoretical idea of friendship further.

- Use scripts and visuals: Using scripts or visual aids can help kids learn conversational skills. A diagram can show how conversations start with introductions and move to deeper topics like hobbies or school subjects. Simple questions like "What's your name?" or "What school do you go to?" can begin the conversation (Chen, 2022). Scripts can help map out conversations, and practicing can develop social skills like responding with "cool" or "thank you."

- Use social stories: Customized stories can teach social skills to kids without coercion. They should match the child's comprehension level and capture their interest.
- Role-playing or behavioral rehearsal: Role-playing or behavioral rehearsal can help kids practice social skills in a safe and structured environment. They can use a specific script or improvise, depending on their needs.
- Use video recording, playing, and editing: Videos can model behaviors and track a child's development. Successful interactions can be recorded and used as future models. Segments of successful actions can be edited together for children who struggle with proper sequence. This is helpful for those who practiced conversational skills separately and need to see them combined into one conversation.

Long-Term Success

Developing social skills takes time, so be patient and plan for the future. Create a timeline for realistic skill development and practice in various environments. Adapt and consider effective approaches. Periodically collect data to track progress and make informed decisions.

KEY POINTS AND TAKEAWAYS

Children with ASD often require assistance to acquire social norms and may experience difficulties with challenging behaviors when interacting with peers. They may need guidance in managing these behaviors and developing positive coping strategies. While friendships and social interactions are crucial for all children, they can be particularly challenging for those with autism, as they may struggle with building and maintaining social skills. Nonetheless, friendships provide a sense of belonging, teach important social skills, and allow children to have fun playing with others.

There are various effective strategies that you can employ to support your child with autism when building friendships. Assimilation strategies can look like helping others understand autism better by providing information. Accommodation involves adapting the social environment to support your child's needs, such as by providing visual aids to help them map out conversations.

It's also essential to teach your child what it means to have a friend—how they should be treated, and how to treat others. This can be done through role-playing and modeling positive social behaviors. Additionally, it's helpful to practice social skills in different environments to improve and refine them. For instance, you can help your child join social groups, participate in community activities, and engage in hobbies that align with their interests. This can provide a natural and supportive setting for children with autism to develop and practice their social skills.

Remember that developing social skills takes time and patience. Be supportive, understanding, and celebratory of any progress their child makes, no matter how small. By implementing these strategies and being persistent, parents can help their child with autism build lasting friendships and develop essential social skills.

This chapter focused on strategies related to Pillar Two, to help you support your child's skill development when it comes to social interactions. In the upcoming section, we will shift our focus to Pillar Four and Pillar Five of the Five Pillar approach. Pillar Four will provide guidance on coping with the stress of caring for a child with autism while maintaining positive relationships with family members despite the challenges. Additionally, Pillar Five offers tips on obtaining financial support to raise a child with ASD and planning for their future.

The forthcoming chapter delves into how autism can impact family life and what parents can do to strengthen their relationships and develop a financial plan for their child. It recognizes that caring for a child with autism can be stressful, and parents may need support to cope with the challenges that come with it.

8

KEEPING THE PEACE AND THE RELATIONSHIPS IN YOUR FAMILY

Motherhood is about raising and celebrating the child you have, not the child you thought you would have. It's about understanding that he is exactly the person he is supposed to be. And that, if you're lucky, he just might be the teacher who turns you into the person you are supposed to be.

— JOAN RYAN

FAMILY MATTERS

Raising a neurodivergent child can be overwhelming, but there are strategies to manage stress and improve relationships. Cognitive reframing, mindfulness, self-care, and seeking professional assistance can help. Respite care, support from family and friends, and financial aid can also be beneficial for families navigating the challenges of raising a child with autism. Care.com provides a comprehensive collection of valuable autism resources for parents and caregivers at:

www.care.com/c/autism-resources-for-parents-and-caregivers.

These approaches align with Pillars Four and Five of the Five Pillar Framework, which provides guidance on managing stress, maintaining healthy family relationships, and finding financial support. It's important to acknowledge that challenges predate the diagnosis and are often a result of societal stigma (Rice, 2021).

AUTISM AND YOUR FAMILY LIFE

An autism diagnosis affects not only the diagnosed child but also their family members. Parents of an autistic child face significant stress from managing therapy schedules, home treatments, and juggling job and family responsibilities, compounded by the financial burden of expensive therapies.

This stress can have adverse effects on family life, and parents of autistic children must navigate the needs of their child and their family. Coping with the challenges of raising an autistic child can strengthen families and marriages, but this requires a robust support system and a lot of hard work.

Parents and Caregivers

According to Psych Central, it's crucial to acknowledge that a diagnosis of autism can significantly impact family life and dynamics (Rice, 2021). This can be a daunting realization, but it doesn't have to be all negative. Family outings, holidays, and traditions can still be enjoyed with some modifications to accommodate your child on the spectrum.

It's important for families to be flexible and make adjustments to help the autistic child feel more comfortable while keeping expectations realistic. This can involve making physical modifications to the environment or changing mindsets and attitudes towards social events. With a little creativity and effort, families can still create plenty of fun memories together.

Don't shy away from activities that may seem challenging or overwhelming. Instead, they should continue to do things together as a family and find ways to adapt activities to meet the needs of everyone involved. By doing so, families can help their child with autism feel included, supported, and valued.

Marriage and Partnerships

After a child is diagnosed with autism, couples may experience challenges in their marriage. They may receive the news differently and struggle to communicate with one another about the diagnosis (Applied Behavior Analysis Programs Guide, n.d.). Additionally, they may have varying expectations on how to manage the changes that come with having a child on the spectrum. Finding time to spend together as a couple can also be challenging, exacerbating an already stressful situation.

To address these issues, couples need to make a concerted effort to prioritize their relationship. This can involve scheduling regular dates to spend alone and reconnecting with one another. It's essential to keep lines of communication open and discuss any concerns or disagreements that arise.

By working together to navigate the unique challenges of raising a child with autism, couples can strengthen their relationship and provide a stable and supportive environment for their child. It takes effort and patience, but with a willingness to communicate and make time for each other, couples can overcome these challenges and grow stronger as a family.

Siblings

Parents may also worry that extra time spent on appointments and behavior management will negatively impact their other children. However, this doesn't necessarily mean the other children will suffer. In fact, they can develop empathy and awareness when parents communicate with them about their sibling's special needs. Family bonds can even become stronger. Remain positive and remember that each family is unique when considering how autism can affect family life.

Finances

Families with an autistic child often face financial challenges as treatments are expensive and not covered by most private health insurance. Studies show they can experience up to a 14% reduction in household income, as both parents struggle to work full-time (Goally, 2021). Losing a job may lead to a loss of health insurance coverage, further impacting the family's finances. Family counseling can help address communication and marital problems, while parents should prioritize their own well-being and not solely focus on the child with autism.

Financial Resource Guide

Raising a child with autism can take a toll on family finances, as medical expenses, therapy sessions, and travel costs can quickly accumulate. To manage this situation effectively, it is crucial to assess your financial situation by calculating your net worth and prioritizing debts. You can explore debt relief options such as negotiating bills, setting up repayment plans, or seeking assistance from support groups. Federal aid programs like Medicaid or flexible spending accounts can help alleviate medical expenses, while charities may offer grants for specific expenses like housing assistance (National Debt Relief, 2022).

Planning for your child's future and independence can be achieved through higher education options, special needs trusts, and emergency funds. The cost of raising a child with special needs may also necessitate relocating to a more suitable area, which could increase costs further. Therefore, budgeting and understanding your financial position are crucial to managing your finances.

When dealing with medical bills, you can request itemized bills, negotiate costs beforehand, or ask for repayment plans. Debt relief and consolidation may also help families struggling with debt. Additionally, several support groups and programs are available to assist families raising children with autism.

Financial Planning

As a parent of a child with autism, it's important to consider their potential level of independence in adulthood when planning your finances. Factors to consider include their position on the spectrum, their ability to obtain higher education, hold a job, and live independently, and the potential need for additional care or services. Once you have a good understanding of this, you can move on to assessing your current net worth by calculating your assets minus liabilities, such as savings accounts, retirement funds, investments, and debts, such as credit cards, student loans, car loans, and mortgages. It's a good idea to use a template to track your net worth and update it quarterly or at least annually.

From there, you can set financial goals for your family, including annual, five-year, and long-term goals. This may include paying off debts, increasing savings, making down payments on a house, paying off student loans, and creating a trust for your child. It's also important to develop a plan to reduce your debts, such as using the debt snowball method or the debt avalanche method, depending on your preference (Hull, 2020).

In addition to debt reduction and savings, you should ensure that both parents have adequate life, health, and disability insurance, as well as business insurance if applicable—this will provide a safety net in case of unforeseen circumstances. It's also important to make sure that your estate is in order with a will, power of attorney, living will, and guardian designation for your children.

Lastly, evaluate your savings plans, including building an emergency fund, saving for college, retirement, and other long-term goals, and consider the type of savings that works best for you, such as a 401(k) or an IRA. By taking all of these steps, you can help secure your family's financial future and provide peace of mind for yourself and your child.

Creating a Financial Plan

It's important to start envisioning a financial plan for your child's adulthood early on. Consider whether your child is interested in and capable of pursuing higher education, whether they can work and earn an income, and if they will be able to live independently. If not, research available living arrangements and review any estate planning already in place, such as a will or trust, to ensure your child is taken care of after you are gone.

Financial Support Options

Numerous financial aid and benefits are available to parents of children with autism, including Supplemental Security Income (SSI), tax credits, Medicaid waivers, 529A accounts, and special needs wills and trusts (Andreasen, 2022). SSI is a form of social security benefit aimed at impoverished families, and the child must have "marked and severe functional limitations" to qualify. Tax benefits include reimbursement of medical expenses and the child and dependent care credit. Medicaid waivers offer support services and care, and 529A accounts allow people with special needs to save money without jeopardizing their eligibility for need-based government assistance. It is important to seek legal advice when creating a special needs will and trust, as gifting money to a child can influence their SSI eligibility.

The Assistive Devices Program (ADP) provides financial support to Ontario residents with long-term physical challenges, covering devices like wheelchairs, hearing aids, and communication aids:

- Financial Assistance: There is financial assistance available to families with autistic children in the United States. The cost of raising a child with ASD can be high, often exceeding $60,000 a year, and the lifetime cost of caring for a child with special needs can range from $1.5 million to $2.4 million (Fay, 2022). However, there are many sources of financial help available, including Supplemental Security Income (SSI), Social Security Survivor Benefits, and VA pensions. SSI provides cash to meet basic needs for food, clothing, and shelter, and eligible children can receive up to $841 per month until they turn 18. Social Security Survivor Benefits may be available to children under 18 or dependent children, and the amount received depends on the parent's average lifetime earnings. VA pensions may provide financial support for dependents and survivors, including minor children and adult children who became disabled before the age of 18. Eligibility for VA pensions doesn't depend on the veteran having a service-related disability.

STRENGTHENING YOUR RELATIONSHIPS

Your Partner

Parenting children with autism has its challenges, but it also has many gifts. Parents who practice strengthening their co-parenting relationship tend to experience less stress and have more positive parenting experiences. These positive effects can then cascade over to all members of the family, including their children.

To strengthen their co-parenting relationship, parents of children with autism can follow some recommendations from a co-parenting training program (Abdullah, 2021). Firstly, they can reflect on their family history and values to identify shared values that connect to their family history and reflect on how they can instill them in their children while adapting to their special needs. Creating a family time capsule and writing a family mission statement can also help summarize this reflection and discussion.

Secondly, co-parents can talk it out by actively listening to each other and avoiding disconfirmation communication. They can also use "I" statements to express their personal needs, plan uninterrupted "check-in" times, and minimize distractions to communicate better.

Thirdly, co-parents can be there for each other by recognizing that working together as a team can reduce their overall stress levels. They can share what increases their stress levels, what they need from one another, and make plans to reduce each other's stress.

Finally, co-parents can use optimism and humor by shifting their perspectives to be more optimistic during check-in times and recognizing how humor can relieve stress. By practicing these recommendations, parents can strengthen their co-parenting relationship, which can have positive effects on all members of the family, including their children.

Children

It can be challenging for neurotypical siblings to build a relationship with their sibling with autism. To help, parents can spend quality time with them and address their concerns when they are frustrated. They can also plan activities that allow their children to enjoy time together and establish family traditions.

Parents should avoid always making their neurotypical child the caregiver for their autistic sibling (Milestones Autism Resources, n.d.). Instead, they can find opportunities for their neurotypical child to engage in age-appropriate activities and spend one-on-one time with them. Parents can also help their children explain their autistic sibling to their friends and provide a comfortable space for their neurotypical child to invite friends over. Additionally, parents can create a special space for their neurotypical child and allow them to have possessions that they do not have to share with their autistic sibling.

To help their autistic child bond with their siblings, parents can highlight their child's strengths and expose them to their neurotypical children's hobbies and interests. Parents can also work on behaviors that may frustrate their neurotypical children and include them when setting priorities for their autistic sibling.

Extended Family

Initially, extended family members may struggle to accept an autism diagnosis due to common stereotypes. While each autistic individual is unique, there are common challenges such as communication difficulties, repetitive behaviors, sensory processing issues, and transition struggles. It's important for them to listen to the parents' diagnosis process and follow evidence-based strategies rather than quick fixes. Supporting an autistic family member involves understanding their challenges and therapy, being flexible during meltdowns and changes in plans, and engaging with them in their interests. For special occasions, it's best to discuss the schedule and ways to engage the child beforehand, provide a quiet space, and be aware of sensory issues (Milestones Autism Resources, n.d.). As a parent, explaining the real issues and seeking help from understanding family members can make a difference. Diplomacy and a focus on symptoms or issues rather than the diagnosis can reduce conflicts with family members who may not understand.

COPING WITH STRESS

When a child is diagnosed with autism, it affects the entire family, but each family member may experience stress in different ways (Raising Children Network Australia, 2017). While some stress can be helpful, too much can be overwhelming and make it hard to manage daily tasks. Therefore, it's important to take steps to manage stress in your family life if you feel that your family is struggling to cope.

Simple Changes

As a parent of an autistic child, start with simple changes to reduce stress. Get enough sleep, exercise, and make time for yourself. Even smaller changes, like slowing down your routine or asking for help, can help. Caring for yourself can benefit your child's functioning too.

Reality

Parents of children with autism may excessively worry about their child's development and future challenges. To manage stress, focus on the present reality and what you can control. Ask, "What is my responsibility to myself and my child today?" (Smith, 2020).

Escape Outside Work

Parents of children with autism often rely on work as a break from caregiving, but it's important for them to have time and space outside of work for self-care. While some may worry about their child's adjustment to a new caregiver, allowing the child to interact with other adults can be beneficial for everyone.

Your Village

Parents of children with ASD experience less stress when they have support systems. Give specific tasks to family and friends who offer help, and point them to resources to learn more. Consider adding organizations, places of worship, schools, and community groups to your support system.

Professionals

Professional help can manage stress levels, even if regular therapy or counseling is not an option. Consider a physician's appointment to ensure good physical health and rule out stress-related complications. Autism organizations, local schools, or hospitals can also connect caregivers with support groups for children on the spectrum, reducing stress and providing valuable resources.

Coping Strategies

Research shows that focusing on seeking help, solving problems, and finding meaning in experiences has better outcomes for parents compared to avoiding emotions and stressors (Johnson, 2021). Social support, whether from family, friends, other ASD families, schools, professionals, or online communities, can also ease parental stress. Other coping mechanisms deemed significant in reducing stress include:

Optimism

To cultivate optimism, shift your thoughts from why things happen to what can be done to change them. For instance, when a favorite service provider leaves, a pessimistic parent may blame themselves for their departure, while an optimistic parent may attribute it to bad luck and focus on helping the next provider be successful (Johnson, 2021). Pessimistic thinking leads to feeling helpless, while optimistic thinking leads to proactive solutions.

Emotional Acceptance

Acceptance is a coping strategy that can reduce parental stress, as comparing an autistic child to non-autistic children can cause anxiety. Recognizing that an autistic child needs specific accommodations, like additional education services and a unique parenting approach, can ease some parental distress.

Cognitive Reframing

Cognitive reframing is a helpful coping technique for families with children who have differences. Parents can see challenging situations as manageable problems instead of blaming the child. This helps them find solutions to the issues.

Mindfulness

Mindfulness programs, including meditation, yoga, physical focus, and thought release, can reduce stress in parents of autistic children, according to studies (Johnson, 2021). These programs also include stressor discussions and light stretching. Parents who participate in them report better sleep, health, and increased self-compassion and well-being, with decreased stress and depression. A study combining mindfulness with positive behavior support training also reduced mothers' stress and aggressive behavior in children (Singh et al., 2019). Parents can improve their health, happiness, and benefit their autistic child and family by recognizing and relieving chronic stress situations.

LEAVING YOUR CHILD

As the parent of a child with autism, taking care of your child can be a daunting task. It's important to establish who will take care of your child and make sure it's someone you trust completely. Our children are vulnerable and need special attention.

Creating a calendar can help with routines and schedules. You may need a monthly, weekly, or daily calendar to keep track of appointments, therapy sessions, and other important events. Having all the necessary phone numbers in an easy-to-see area of your home is also important. Write down any numbers that may be important, such as doctors, therapists, or emergency contacts.

Make sure to have a necessary medication list and schedule. Include any vitamins and medications your child needs, along with the times and amounts they need to be taken. Talking to your child about what will happen is also crucial. Kids with autism thrive on routines and schedules, so it's essential to go over any changes with your child, repeat them, and remind them of them to make the transition easier (Nedeoglo, 2019).

SUPPORT GROUPS

Support groups are invaluable for parents of children with autism. They offer an inclusive and non-judgmental space for sharing experiences and coping strategies. Confidentiality is ensured, and support groups can also provide information about available resources and help parents become advocates for their children. Through support groups, parents can gain a better understanding of autism and feel more confident in their ability to make informed decisions about their child's care. This community of individuals understands the unique challenges faced by parents of autistic children.

There are numerous support groups available to parents of children with autism that offer a platform for connection, resources, and advocacy. The Autism Support Group and the Autism Society provide various resources and support to families affected by autism. Parenting Autism offers online forums, educational resources, and a network of parents and caregivers who can empathize with the challenges of raising a child with autism. Autism Now provides information on autism services and support for individuals and families. MyAutismTeam is a social network that allows parents to connect with others, share advice and support, and access resources. Lastly, Dads 4 Special Kids is a support group specifically for fathers of children with special needs, including autism, offering resources, networking opportunities, and a safe space for fathers to share their experiences and connect with others in similar situations.

There are many Facebook groups available for parents and individuals affected by autism and related conditions. These groups provide a supportive community and resources for managing the challenges of autism. The Autism and Asperger's Syndrome Support Group is one such group, offering a space for individuals impacted by autism and Asperger's syndrome to connect and share their experiences.

Parenting Asperger's Children is a group specifically for parents of children with Asperger's syndrome, while Parenting Defiant Children and Teens offer support and resources for parents dealing with defiant behavior in their children, including those with autism. There are also Facebook groups geared towards parents of high-functioning autistic children, including Parenting High-Functioning Autistic Children and Parenting Children With Level 1 Autism.

Facebook also offers several groups for partners and spouses of those on the autism spectrum, including Relationships with Asperger's Spouses and Partners, Relationships With Partners On The Autism Spectrum, and Women in Relationships with Asperger's Men.

For adults with Asperger's and high-functioning autism, there are Facebook groups, such as Adults with Asperger's and High-Functioning Autism, which offer a supportive community and resources for managing life with these conditions. Lastly, Support for Women on the Autism Spectrum is a group specifically for women with autism to connect and share their experiences.

KEY POINTS AND TAKEAWAYS

After reading this chapter, you will be better equipped to manage financial stress and improve relationships when raising a child with autism. Seek financial support and use available programs to help with expenses related to therapy, education, and medical care. Strategies to improve family relationships include involving siblings in therapy and addressing conflicts with extended family members. Remember that raising a child with autism can bring families closer together. This chapter focused on Pillars Four and

Five of the Five Pillar Framework, which provides guidance on managing stress, maintaining strong family relationships, and finding financial support. The final chapter will explore methods for promoting character development and improving skills for a successful future.

9

HELPING YOUR CHILD THRIVE

Kids have to be exposed to different things in order to develop. A kid's not going to find out he likes to play a musical instrument if you never exposed him to it.

— TEMPLE GRANDIN

THRIVE, NOT SURVIVE

In this chapter, we will delve into strategies that parents can use to assist their children on the autism spectrum in discovering and developing their inherent potential, with the aim of setting them up for success in life. This chapter is aligned with Pillar Two of the

Five Pillar framework, which focuses on fostering character growth, unlocking inherent potential, and enhancing abilities. By leveraging their strengths, parents can help their children reach their full potential while also addressing their challenges in a supportive and positive way.

Some of the strategies that will be explored in this chapter include identifying the child's unique strengths and interests, providing opportunities for exploration and growth, setting achievable goals, and celebrating successes along the way. By nurturing the inherent potential of children with ASD, parents can help them overcome their challenges and achieve their goals. This not only improves their quality of life but also empowers them to become successful individuals who can contribute positively to society. Through these strategies, parents can unlock their children's unique gifts and talents, helping them reach their full potential and achieve success in their personal and professional lives.

IQ OVER TIME

A recent study by researchers at the MIND Institute of the University of California, Davis, reveals that intelligence levels in autistic children between the ages of 2 and 8 years old do not remain stable (Solomon et al., 2017). The study examined the IQ scores of 102 children, including 20 girls, at 2 or 3 years old, and then again at ages 6 to 8. Based on their IQ changes, the children were grouped into four categories: two showed IQ improvements, while the other two showed steady or decreasing IQs. A total of 55% of the children experienced IQ gains as they grew older, leading to reduced internalizing and externalizing behaviors over time. However, the study was limited in scope, as it did not include children from low-income or rural areas, and thus may not reflect a wider national trend. The study also found that the separate groups presented distinct patterns of change in communication skills and autism severity.

Giftedness

Giftedness is characterized by extraordinary ability, a high IQ, or both, leading to a different way of experiencing the world. Gifted children exhibit unique characteristics such as faster learning, acute memory, and increased complexity in thinking and reasoning. An IQ score of 130 or higher is considered gifted, but cognitive assessments beyond IQ tests are needed for identification. Giftedness and academic achievement are not the same, and a gifted student may struggle in school if they lack interest or are anxious, frustrated, or depressed. Gifted children may experience lower grades if early education is too easy, leading to a lack of study skills and work ethic. Gifted students have uneven development and greater emotional sensitivity than high achievers. Some gifted programs may include high achievers, but not necessarily gifted students based on achievement criteria.

Intelligence and Autism

One in 59 children in the US have autism, with 70% having an intellectual disability, or an IQ lower than 70 (Lovering, 2021). The remaining 30% have intelligence ranging from average to gifted, as autism and intelligence are separate characteristics. However, some traits are common between giftedness and autism, such as idealism, intense focus, high learning drive, sensory differences, vivid imagination, difficulty sitting still, challenges with emotional regulation, niche expertise, and logical/precise, and divergent thinking.

Twice Exceptional

Twice exceptional, or 2e, refers to individuals who have both intellectual giftedness and a neurobiological difference, motor skills issue, or learning disability such as autism, dyslexia, ADHD, or dyspraxia (Lovering, 2021). While giftedness and autism are separate traits, giftedness can compensate for other issues but also intensify them, which may cause barriers to diagnosis and delay support.

IDENTIFYING TALENT

Autistic children may find it difficult to develop language and motor skills, which can be discouraging for their parents who want them to progress like their peers. However, it is important to have patience and explore alternative avenues to uncover their hidden talents. Evidence suggests that having an autism diagnosis doesn't mean a child can't achieve great things. Finding these talents might require unconventional methods, but with perseverance, it is possible to encourage an autistic child to flourish.

Interest

As a parent of an autistic child who has been formally diagnosed, it is crucial to observe their activities and interests to discover possible talents. Often, their obsessions can be indicative of hidden talents. It is beneficial to encourage and develop these abilities, as it can enhance the child's morale as well as that of the caregiver.

Discovering your child's interests and abilities can assist them in job hunting. As an illustration, my grandson possesses exceptional computer skills and is proficient in sorting and organizing; thus, cell phone repair would be an excellent occupation for him. Presently, he volunteers at a library and sorts and re-shelves books. Additionally, he has a paying job with a non-profit where he prepares items to be sold by sorting and pricing them. Due to his impressive concentration skills, he can work for several hours, and both he and his employers enjoy the job.

Assessment

In ABA therapy, therapists observe a child's behavior, emotions, and other unspoken activities to find the most effective approach (Morrison, 2021). They analyze the child's behavior in various settings, identifying triggers and outcomes. They also look for latent talents that can be developed and collaborate with parents to create a treatment plan. The child's strengths in certain areas may be communicated to schools.

Treatment

Early treatment benefits autistic children by uncovering hidden talents. Therapists work with parents to create individualized plans based on each child's unique strengths and needs. Building confidence and independence takes time and patience. ABA therapists may encourage parents to support their child's evolving interests, such as art or sports (Morrison, 2021).

Exposure and Experience

Autistic children can find alternative ways to express themselves through art and other forms of expression. With the right tools and support, they can pursue their interests and communicate their preferences.

Interpretations

The exposure of autistic children to art forms such as music and visual art can enhance their independent thinking and interpretation abilities. ABA therapists can help parents identify their child's strengths and niches, thus promoting interpretation and exploration (Morrison, 2021).

Fun Sensory Activities

Engaging children in sensory activities can be a great way to encourage self-expression and exploration. Finger and footprint painting, making slime, and scented playdough are some examples of sensory activities that can provide a supersensory experience. For outdoor activities, a mud kitchen can be an excellent choice where children can create and experiment using mud, water, bowls, and various utensils (Foster Care Associates, 2022). Creating musical instruments, a sensory ocean with sand and water, painting with food, and toys in jelly can also be enjoyable for children. Another idea is to set up a pouring station with different-sized bottles, jugs, cups, and containers to encourage children to pour water from one container to another, learn fine motor skills, and mix colors. These activities can be a great way to engage children and encourage their development.

CHANGING SCHOOLS

The U.S. Department of Education states that all children, regardless of their abilities, have the right to receive a free education in an environment that is not overly restrictive (Sarah Dooley Center for Autism, 2018). For children with autism, this may mean transitioning from an autism-specific school to a mainstream school for some or all of their day. However, parents may feel anxious about whether their child is ready to thrive in a different academic environment without the specialized support offered by the autism school.

It's important to know that educators carefully evaluate each child's abilities and coping skills before making a recommendation to transition from an autism school to a mainstream school.

Assessment Areas

Academic

To attend school, a child must be academically prepared and evaluated by educators on their ability to comprehend coursework, study, meet expectations, adjust to teaching styles, and be on track with peers. Educators evaluate placement options if there are academic gaps to ensure the child can fit in academically. The child's grade level matters, and they must handle grade-specific demands before switching schools. While catching up is common, evaluating academic gaps is important for success in the new school.

Emotional

Moving to a new school involves many changes for a child, such as different transportation, academic challenges, and new peers and teachers. The evaluation team will assess the child's problem-solving skills, resilience, and ability to handle and embrace change when evaluating their readiness for this transition.

Behavioral

To transition to a mainstream environment, a child with autism must demonstrate the ability to handle the new school without negative behaviors. Accommodations like fidget tools and physical movement may be allowed, but the child must possess coping skills and appropriate behavior to ensure a calm and safe environment for everyone.

Social

Before transitioning to a mainstream school, a child with autism must be prepared to handle the different social environment, including large class sizes, crowded hallways, and different social expectations. This involves understanding and exhibiting acceptable social behavior, managing bullying, making friends, and controlling impulses. These social skills demonstrate to educators that the child is ready for the transition, although social development will continue to occur over time.

Communication

To transition successfully to a mainstream environment, a child needs good communication skills to interact with peers and teachers. It is essential for them to advocate for themselves, participate in discussions, ask for help, and read nonverbal cues to navigate the new school environment.

Independence

A child in mainstream school must be fairly independent, as there is limited teacher assistance. An aide or Personal Care Assistant may be provided through their Individualized Education Program, but the child will primarily navigate the school independently, with educators ensuring they can handle academic, social, and behavioral demands.

Alternative Options

When transitioning a child with autism to a mainstream school, their readiness and needs should be assessed. A full-time or gradual transition may be appropriate, and there are various options to ease them into the new environment. These include attending a larger class size in the autism school, taking a mainstream art, physical education, or math class, joining an inclusion class, and receiving academic and emotional support like an aide, tutor, or occupational therapist. Collaboration with educators and support teams is essential to determining the best approach for the child's unique needs and abilities.

Transitioning

The child's coping skills and abilities are evaluated by educators to determine their readiness for transitioning from an autism school to a mainstream school. It's crucial to share your own observations and insights when selecting a school environment that would encourage your child with autism to learn, grow and succeed in the future.

Advocating for Your Child

Advocating for your autistic child at school can be challenging. To be effective, Dr. Emma Goodall, an autism consultant, recommends being positive and constructive, asking about support plans and communication support, being flexible and realistic, establishing clear communication with teachers, and providing a concise sensory support plan (Churchman & Saunders, 2019). Focus on what teachers need to know about your child rather than a lengthy analysis.

TRANSITION TO ADOLESCENCE

Parents of teenagers with autism spectrum disorder (ASD) may wonder how the physical and hormonal changes of adolescence will affect their child. Research is still limited, but some changes can be expected, such as improvements in daily living skills and behavioral improvements. However, there may be more challenges during adolescence, such as the onset of seizures, anxiety, and executive functioning problems. Executive functioning is the ability to plan, remember past experiences, work in groups, maintain self-control, and change course if necessary. Teens with ASD tend to mature at a slower pace in executive skills, which can create problems in high school when the demands on teens increase dramatically. Schools and parents can help by providing external support to the teen, such as frequent parent-school communication and breaking down complex projects into smaller steps.

Teenage Thriving

Raising a teenager with autism can be challenging due to the significant changes that come with adolescence. To help your child thrive during this time, encourage independence, foster social skills, encourage communication, prepare for changes, and encourage positive self-esteem. Teenagers with autism may have difficulty communicating and establishing relationships, leading to isolation and increased anxiety and depression. However, with ABA therapy and support from parents and caregivers, they can develop skills to interact successfully with their peers (ABA Centers of America, 2022). Seek help from professionals, keep communication open, and focus on their strengths. With the right support system, teenagers with autism can overcome challenges and participate in their communities.

Productive Young Adults

The milestones that individuals with ASD should aim for as they grow older will vary based on their individual needs. For those with severe developmental delays, positive outcomes can include integration into school and community environments by age 6, the development of adaptive functioning skills, reduced levels of needed support, and forming social connections. For those with milder delays, successful outcomes may include thriving in mainstream classrooms, building a community network, and requiring limited additional support for more complex social situations. Goals for adults and adolescents with severe developmental struggles may include functioning with community support, minimizing aggressive behavior, contributing to vocational opportunities, and achieving semi-autonomous living. Meanwhile, those with milder delays may strive for relationships and friendships, success in school and work, a lower risk of mental health issues, and limited therapy needs. With the right support and treatment, individuals with ASD can succeed in almost any career.

Independent Living

Parents of children with autism can take several steps to nurture their child's independence and help them lead a fulfilling life. Firstly, connecting with local parent groups such as Matrix, the Autism Society of America, and Autism Speaks can provide valuable resources and information on innovative residential projects (Kaplan, 2021). Taking a leadership role in these meetings can be especially helpful. Secondly, it is essential to lay a strong foundation by nurturing independence from the very beginning. Parents can encourage their child to participate in daily activities such as dressing themselves, putting clothes in the laundry hamper, sorting clothes, picking out their clothing, and putting the clothing away after it has been washed. Children can also be taught to strip and make the bed, set the table, take finished dishes to the sink, and load the dishwasher. As children grow, parents can gradually increase their responsibilities, such as taking them shopping and gradually increasing the number of items they need to find. Other activities that can promote independence include teaching children how to replace light bulbs, participating in bathing or showering, and following a checklist of steps for washing and rinsing their bodies. By taking these steps, parents can help their children develop the skills and confidence they need to become independent adults.

STORIES

Despite the challenges that people with ASD may face, including difficulty communicating and maintaining friendships, obsessive interests, and delayed speech, these 15 individuals have not let those challenges get in the way of achieving their dreams. These business leaders, intellectuals, artists, and other highly successful people with autism have inspired millions of people, and their stories are sure to inspire you too (Skibitsky, n.d.).

Dr. Temple Grandin

Temple Grandin is a highly inspiring individual—despite being diagnosed with autism as a child and remaining non-verbal until three-and-a-half years of age, she learned to speak with the help of a speech therapist and went on to write Emergence: Labeled Autistic, a groundbreaking book that offered insight into the life and thoughts of a person with autism. Dr. Grandin is a prolific writer and speaker who focuses on both autism and animal behavior. She is currently a Professor of Animal Science at Colorado

University and has been named "the most accomplished and well-known adult with autism in the world." In 2010, Time Magazine named her one of the 100 most influential people in the world, and her life was the subject of a biographical film starring Claire Danes, who won an Emmy Award for her portrayal.

Wolfgang Amadeus Mozart

Mozart likely showed signs of Tourettes and Asperger's, according to experts who retrospectively diagnosed him. These traits did not affect his creativity or hinder his progress. He composed over 600 pieces and is widely considered one of the greatest composers in history, with many of his works still regarded as classical music's finest examples.

Satoshi Tajiri

Satoshi Tajiri, diagnosed with Asperger's Syndrome, created Pokémon by combining his love for insect collecting and Nintendo's Game Boy. The franchise has become the most successful media franchise, valued at $15 billion, with games, books, movies, and merchandise. Tajiri confirmed his Asperger's diagnosis but prefers to let his work speak for itself.

Emily Dickinson

Emily Dickinson, a renowned poet, may have been on the autism spectrum, according to Julie Brown's book, "Writers on the Spectrum." Dickinson's epilepsy is well-known, but her quirky behaviors and characteristics are also attributed to autism.

Anthony Ianni

Anthony Ianni was diagnosed with PDD-NOS (Pervasive Developmental Disorder—Not Otherwise Specified, formerly a subtype of autism) and told by doctors that he would not achieve much in life. But he used this prediction as motivation to achieve great things, becoming the first person with autism to play First Division basketball and winning the NCAA National Championship with the Michigan Spartans in 2000. Today, he is a motivational speaker who encourages young people with autism to pursue their dreams without limitations.

Sir Anthony Hopkins

Sir Anthony Hopkins, the Oscar-winning star of The Silence of the Lambs and other classic movies, has openly discussed being diagnosed with high-functioning Asperger's. Despite genuinely liking people, he revealed in an interview that being on the spectrum has resulted in having fewer friends and attending fewer parties. Nevertheless, Sir Anthony has become one of the most successful actors of his generation and is beloved by millions.

Albert Einstein

Einstein needs no introduction, as he is one of the most successful people with autism. He developed the theory of relativity, E=MC2, and is widely regarded as one of the most influential scientists of his generation. However, not everyone knows that he met many criteria for autism. He didn't speak until he was three years old, then immediately spoke in complete sentences. His inflexible insistence on routines and difficulty with people led many analysts to believe he would have been diagnosed with ASD if tested during his lifetime.

Dani Bowman

Dani Bowman has been inspiring fellow young people on the autism spectrum from a young age, unlike others who wait until adulthood. She is a talented illustrator and animator who founded her own company, DaniMation Entertainment, at the age of 11 and began working in the animation industry at 14. Bowman is a passionate autism advocate and public speaker who encourages people with ASD and disabilities to reach their full potential, follow their dreams, and achieve their goals.

Andy Warhol

Andy Warhol, known for his eccentricity and pop art, was never diagnosed with autism. However, many experts believe he displayed autism-like characteristics, such as social ineptness and difficulty recognizing friends. He used few words in his speech and insisted on routine and uniformity. Most experts suggest he had Asperger's, but it didn't stop him from becoming an iconic artist.

Daryl Hannah

Daryl Hannah, known for her roles in blockbuster movies like Blade Runner, Wall Street, and Steel Magnolias, has discussed in interviews how her Asperger's syndrome diagnosis affected her career. She has expressed feeling socially awkward and uncomfortable at premieres and events, and how her behavior due to her Asperger's had led her to feel "practically blacklisted" from the movie industry. However, Hannah persevered and continued to succeed, appearing in critically acclaimed movies like Kill Bill as well as other popular films and theater productions.

Dan Aykroyd

Dan Aykroyd, a Canadian performer, has publicly disclosed that he was diagnosed with both Tourette's and Asperger's as a child. He has attributed his fixation on ghosts, which stems from the obsessive traits of autism, as the inspiration for creating the Ghostbusters movie.

Susan Boyle

Susan Boyle's appearance on the UK TV show Britain's Got Talent was initially met with ridicule due to her shy and awkward appearance. However, her stunning voice silenced her naysayers and won over the audience. Boyle's subsequent career saw her sell over 14 million albums, perform sold-out concerts, and gain a devoted following, all while living with Asperger's Syndrome, a diagnosis she found to be a "relief" as it helped her understand and accept her uniqueness.

Clay Marzo

Clay Marzo, despite being diagnosed with Asperger's Syndrome, became one of the most innovative and influential stars in championship surfing. He won swimming competitions as a child and finished third in the National Scholastic Surfing Association (NSSA) Nationals at 11 years old, which led to him signing with the Quicksilver team. Four years later, he became the first surfer to achieve two perfect 10s in NSSA history and won the national championship. Marzo starred in the documentary "Clay Marzo: Just Add Water," where he talked about his accomplishments and his experience with Asperger's. He currently volunteers with Surfers Healing, a charity that teaches young people with autism how to surf.

Tony DeBlois

Tony DeBlois, who was born blind, started playing the piano when he was only two years old, displaying a natural talent for the instrument. However, his abilities were not limited to just the piano. Despite being diagnosed with autism, he has mastered more than 20 instruments and can perform up to 8,000 pieces of music entirely from memory. DeBlois has released several albums, toured globally, and was the subject of a television movie based on his life.

Dr. Vernon Smith

Dr. Vernon Smith, a pioneering economics professor, is credited with inventing experimental economics, which led to his 2002 Nobel Prize in Economic Sciences. He has been open about his Asperger's syndrome and attributes much of his success to his autism, saying that he feels no social pressure to conform to the way others approach problems in economics.

KEY POINTS AND TAKEAWAYS

In the final chapter of our book, we focused on Pillar Two of the Five Pillar framework, which provides parents with practical strategies for helping their child with ASD discover their potential and nurture their gifts for success. We offered tips on finding the right educational program, preparing for the transition to adulthood, and developing life skills and job training. Embracing our child's unique characteristics and appreciating their strengths is key. We shared inspiring stories of successful people on the autism spectrum to showcase their boundless potential with adequate support and guidance. Our aim is to equip parents with the necessary resources to recognize and maximize their child's capabilities, as every child has incredible potential.

Your Chance to Help Another Parent

With the Five Pillar Framework by your side, you're better prepared for every challenge ahead of you – and that puts you in the perfect position to help other parents.

Simply by sharing your honest opinion of this book on Amazon, you'll show new readers where they can find all the guidance they need to feel confident in their ability to support their child.

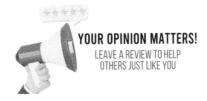

YOUR OPINION MATTERS!
LEAVE A REVIEW TO HELP
OTHERS JUST LIKE YOU

Thank you for your support… Let's spread this information far and wide!

Scan the QR code to leave review!

CONCLUSION

As a guide for parents with children who have ASD or Asperger's syndrome, this resource offers a comprehensive overview and covers a range of difficult topics that can help parents understand their child. This includes how to communicate with loved ones about their diagnosis, how to support children with ASD in their social interactions and communication, ways to handle repetitive behaviors and obsessions, how to address sensory problems and sleep issues, and how to manage aggressive behavior and discipline ASD children.

In addition, the guide provides advice on socialization and making friends for children with ASD, how autism affects family life, and how parents can prepare financially for their child's future. There are also practical tips for planning education and finances, as well as strategies for helping children transition into adulthood and live independently.

We have featured motivational accounts of real individuals who have autism, including acquaintances, coworkers, and well-known successful figures. These narratives highlight the distinctive strengths and capabilities of children who are diagnosed with ASD and underscore the significance of nurturing their aptitudes and supporting them in realizing their maximum potential in life.

All of this information revolves around a 360-degree, Five Pillar approach. These Five Pillars are meant to address a specific aspect of parenting children with Autism Spectrum Disorder (ASD) and Asperger's syndrome, and each chapter corresponds to a different pillar, or sometimes even a combination of them.

Pillar One aims to provide insights into why children with ASD behave the way they do. This helps parents understand their child's condition and implement effective strategies discussed in Pillar Two to foster character growth and unlock their potential. Pillar Three covers tactics for handling unpredictable behavior, including obsessive and hostile conduct, and addressing sensory challenges. Pillar Four outlines methods for managing the stress of caring for an autistic child while maintaining healthy family relationships. Lastly, Pillar Five provides suggestions for obtaining financial assistance and preparing for the future, helping parents provide the best support for their child with ASD.

Your child with autism is a unique individual with their own special talents and gifts. While they may approach the world differently than others, it's important to remember that all children have their own quirks and differences. Focus on your child's strengths, interests, and abilities to help them reach their full potential and live a happy and healthy life.

By implementing the strategies outlined in the Five Pillar framework, you can effectively support your child with autism and help them thrive. You can now better understand and respond to their behavior, encourage their social and emotional development, manage their sensory challenges, and create a positive and supportive environment at home. Additionally, you can plan for your child's financial future while handling stress and maintaining healthy relationships with your family.

Remember that your child is not defined by their diagnosis and has limitless potential. With your support and guidance, they can overcome obstacles and achieve great things. Embrace their unique perspectives and strengths, and watch them flourish into the amazing person they were always meant to be.

REFERENCES

4 Ways Autism Causes Stress in the Family. (2021, June 24). Goally. https://getgoally.com/blog/4-ways-autism-impact-the-family/

11 Tips on How to Design a Room for Kids with Autism. (2021, March 29). Magical Nest. https://magicalnest.com/blogs/news/11-tips-on-how-to-design-a-room-for-kids-with-autism

10 Fun Sensory Activities for a Child with Autism. (2022). Foster Care Associates. https://www.thefca.co.uk/fostering-autistic-children/sensory-activities-children-autism/

A quote by Amanda Rae Ross. (n.d.). People's Care. https://peoplescare.com/amazing-autism-quotes/

A quote by Claire LaZebnik. (n.d.). Overall Motivation. https://www.overallmotivation.com/quotes/autism-quotes/

A quote by Joan Ryan. (n.d.). Goodreads. https://www.goodreads.com/quotes/345624-motherhood-is-about-raising-and-celebrating-the-child-you-have

A quote by Lyndon B. Johnson. (n.d.). BrainyQuote. https://www.brainyquote.com/quotes/lyndon_b_johnson_103549

A quote by Temple Grandin. (n.d.-a). Cross River Therapy. https://www.crossrivertherapy.com/autism/quotes

A quote by Temple Grandin. (n.d.-b). Hidden Talents ABA. https://hiddentalentsaba.com/autism-quotes/

A quote by Tricia Goyer. (n.d.). Goodreads. https://www.goodreads.com/work/quotes/61651624-calming-angry-kids-help-and-hope-for-parents-in-the-whirlwind

A quote by Unknown. (n.d.). Youth Dynamics. https://www.youthdynamics.org/18-quotes-to-help-you-on-the-path-to-purposeful-parenting/

A quote by Violet Stevens. (n.d.). Autism Parenting Magazine. https://www.autismparentingmagazine.com/quotes-about-autism/

A quote by Yoda. (n.d.). Successful Spirit. https://www.thesuccessfulspirit.com/in-a-dark-place-we-find-ourselves/

Abdullah, M. (2021, February 19). *How Parents of Children With Autism Can*

Strengthen Their Relationship. Greater Good Magazine. https://greatergood. berkeley.edu/article/item/ how_parents_of_children_with_autism_can_strengthen_their_relation ship

Aggression & Autism: How to Manage Aggressive Behavior. (2022, February 3). Behavioral Innovations - ABA Therapy for Kids with Autism. https:// behavioral-innovations.com/blog/aggression-in-children-with-autism/

Aggression in Autism - One Simple Cause. (2021, July 24). Thinking Autism Taking Action. https://www.thinkingautism.org.uk/aggression-in-autism-one-simple-cause/

Anderson, C. (2015, November 11). *Children With Autism and Aggression.* SPARK for Autism. https://sparkforautism.org/discover_article/children-with-autism-and-aggression/

Andreasen, H. (2022, April 2). *Can I get financial assistance for my autistic child? | Autism Resources.* Songbird Therapy. https://www.songbirdcare.com/arti cles/can-i-get-financial-assistance-for-my-child-with-autism

Autism. (2022, March 29). World Health Organization (WHO). https://www. who.int/news-room/fact-sheets/detail/autism-spectrum-disorders

Autism communication strategies. (2021, October 25). LeafWing Center. https:// leafwingcenter.org/autism-communication-strategies/

Autism Spectrum Disorder. (2022, March). National Institute of Mental Health. https://www.nimh.nih.gov/health/topics/autism-spectrum-disorders-asd

Barbera, M. (2022, March 29). *Why Timeouts Don't Work and Alternatives You Can Use Instead.* Dr. Mary Barbera. https://marybarbera.com/why-time outs-dont-work-alternatives/

Barloso, K. (2019, July 29). *Autism Social Skills: How to Enhance Social Interaction.* Autism Parenting Magazine. https://www.autismparenting magazine.com/autism-social-skills/

Beversdorf, D. (2014, July). *How to Get Tested for Autism as an Adult.* Autism Speaks. https://www.autismspeaks.org/expert-opinion/getting-evalu ated-autism-adult-where-go-who-see

Broady, T. R., Stoyles, G. J., & Morse, C. (2015). Understanding carers' lived experience of stigma: the voice of families with a child on the autism spec-trum. *Health & Social Care in the Community, 25*(1), 224–233. https://doi. org/10.1111/hsc.12297

Burtt, K. (2022, February 22). *18 Celebrities Who Have Opened Up About Raising a Kid With a Disability*. DIVERSEability Magazine. https://diverseability magazine.com/2022/02/18-celebrities-opened-raising-kid-disability/

Carmen B. Pingree Autism Center of Learning. (2021, February 18). *Sensitivity Differences In Autism: Sensory Overload*. The Carmen B. Pingree Autism Center of Learning. https://carmenbpingree.com/blog/sensory-overload-in-autism/

Chen, G. (2022). *Helping Children with Autism Develop Friendships*. Stages Learning. https://blog.stageslearning.com/blog/helping-children-with-autism-develop-friendship

Churchman, F. (2019, April 9). *Strategies for helping autistic children (and their families) get a good night's sleep*. ABC Everyday. https://www.abc.net.au/everyday/how-to-help-children-with-autism-get-a-good-nights-sleep/10974346

Churchman, F., & Saunders, T. (2019, April 1). *Being the best advocate for your autistic child at school*. ABC Everyday. https://www.abc.net.au/everyday/being-the-best-advocate-for-your-autistic-child-at-school/10947344

Communicating with a child who has Aspergers? (2021, December 20). SpecialKids.company. https://ca.specialkids.company/blogs/latest-news/communicating-with-a-child-who-has-aspergers?shpxid=da8a3c20-5f17-48a7-9058-f5e5a690fb64

Communication: autistic children. (2021, May 19). Raising Children Network Australia. https://raisingchildren.net.au/autism/communicating-relation ships/communicating/communication-asd

Cooperman, T. (n.d.). *Autism Supplements - Which are Beneficial for Autism?* ConsumerLab.com. Retrieved April 23, 2023, from https://www.consumerlab.com/answers/which-supplements-have-been-shown-to-be-helpful-for-autism/supplements-for-autism/

Creating a Long-Term Financial Plan for Your Child with Autism. (2021, November 5). American Advocacy Group. https://www.americanadvoca cygroup.com/creating-a-long-term-financial-plan-for-your-child-with-autism/

Deolinda, A. (2021, April 8). *Center Stage: Famous People With Autism*. Autism Parenting Magazine. https://www.autismparentingmagazine.com/famous-people-with-autism/

Dietert, R. R., Dietert, J. M., & Dewitt, J. C. (2011). Environmental risk factors for autism. *Emerging Health Threats Journal*, *4*(1), 7111. https://doi.org/10.

3402/ehtj.v4i0.7111

Discipline strategies for autistic children and teenagers. (2020b, November 18). Raising Children Network Australia. https://raisingchildren.net.au/autism/behaviour/common-concerns/discipline-for-children-teens-with-asd

Divine Academy. *(2020, July 2). 20 great quotes about autism and special needs.* divineacademy. https://www.divineacademy.com/post/20-great-quotes-about-autism-and-special-needs

Drake, K. (2021, July 29). *Elon Musk Opened Up About Autism: Here's What We Learned.* Psych Central. https://psychcentral.com/autism/elon-musk-opened-up-about-autism-heres-what-we-learned#response-to-musk

Ebert, M. (2022). *Strategies for Responding to Rude Comments About Your Child's Behavior.* Stages Learning. https://blog.stageslearning.com/blog/strategies-for-responding-to-rude-comments-about-your-childs-behavior

Family stress and autism spectrum disorder. (2017, January 31). Raising Children Network Australia. https://raisingchildren.net.au/autism/communicating-relationships/family-relationships/family-stress-asd

Fay, M. (2022, August 26). *Financial Help for Special Needs Children & Their Families.* Debt.org. https://www.debt.org/advice/financial-help-special-needs/

Financial Resource Guide For Families Of Children With Autism. (2022, November 21). National Debt Relief. https://www.nationaldebtrelief.com/financial-resource-guide-for-families-of-children-with-autism/

Gailliot, M. T., & Baumeister, R. F. (2007). The Physiology of Willpower: Linking Blood Glucose to Self-Control. *Personality and Social Psychology Review, 11*(4), 303–327. https://doi.org/10.1177/1088868307303030

Goldwert, L. (2012, June 5). *Tommy Hilfiger: My daughter Kathleen, wife Dee's son both on autism spectrum.* New York Daily News. https://www.nydailynews.com/life-style/health/tommy-hilfiger-daughter-kathleen-wife-dee-son-autism-spectrum-article-1.1089738

Gray, D. E. (1993). Perceptions of stigma: the parents of autistic children. *Sociology of Health and Illness, 15*(1), 102–120. https://doi.org/10.1111/1467-9566.ep11343802

Gray, D. E. (2002). "Everybody just freezes. Everybody is just embarrassed": felt and enacted stigma among parents of children with high functioning autism. *Sociology of Health & Illness*, *24*(6), 734–749. https://doi.org/10. 1111/1467-9566.00316

Hargitai, L., Livingston, L. A., & Shah, P. (2022, November 14). *Elon Musk: how being autistic may make him think differently*. The Conversation. https:// theconversation.com/elon-musk-how-being-autistic-may-make-him-think-differently-194228

How do I tell people my child has autism? A complete guide to hard conversations. (2023, March 28). Beaming Health. https://beaminghealth.com/article/how-do-i-tell-people-my-child-has-autism

How Does Autism Affect Family Life? (n.d.). Applied Behavior Analysis Programs Guide. https://www.appliedbehavioranalysisprograms.com/faq/how-does-autism-affect-family-life/

How to Deal with Obsessive and Repetitive Behaviour. (2023a). Durham Region Autism Services. https://www.durham-autism.org/obsessive-repetitive-behaviour-autism/

How to Improve Listening Skills in Children with ADHD and Autism. (2018, December 21). Special Strong. https://www.specialstrong.com/how-to-improve-listening-skills-in-children-with-adhd-and-autism/

How to Move From An Autism School To A Mainstream School. (2018, February 28). Sarah Dooley Center for Autism. https://www.sarahdooleycenter. org/news/how-to-move-from-an-autism-school-to-a-mainstream-school/

Hull, T. (2020, December 24). *Essential Financial Planning: 10 considerations for families with an autistic child*. Autism & ADHD Connection. https:// autismadhdconnection.com/essential-financial-planning-10-considera tions-for-families-with-an-autistic-child/

Jewell, T. (2020, April 16). *Asperger's vs. Autism: What's the Difference?* Healthline. https://www.healthline.com/health/aspergers-vs-autism#about-aspergers

Johnson, K. (2021, May 20). *How Parents and Caregivers of Kids with Autism Cope with Stress*. LEARN Behavioral. https://learnbehavioral.com/blog/how-parents-and-caregivers-of-kids-with-autism-cope-with-stress

Kanne, S. M., & Mazurek, M. O. (2010). Aggression in Children and Adolescents with ASD: Prevalence and Risk Factors. *Journal of Autism and Developmental Disorders*, *41*(7), 926–937. https://doi.org/10.1007/s10803-010-1118-4

Kaplan, K. (2021, January 29). *How to Prepare your Autistic Child for Independent Living.* Autism Parenting Magazine. https://www.autismparenting magazine.com/asd-independent-living/

King, H. (2022, April 15). *Elon Musk opens up about growing up with Asperger's.* Axios. https://www.axios.com/2022/04/15/elon-musk-aspergers-syndrome

Lee, K. (2022, December 5). *Reasons Why Time Out May Not Be Working for Your Child.* Verywell Family. https://www.verywellfamily.com/reasons-why-time-out-may-not-be-working-for-your-child-3858981

Loiselle, M. (2021, April 2). *How to Explain Autism to Children.* Indy's Child Magazine. https://indyschild.com/how-to-explain-autism-to-children/#:~:text=%E2%80%9CFor%20an%20even%20younger%20child

Lovering, N. (2021, October 26). *Giftedness and Autism: What to Know.* Psych Central. https://psychcentral.com/autism/autistic-and-gifted-supporting-the-twice-exceptional-child

Marks, J. L. (2018, August 29). *Does My Child Have Asperger's Syndrome or Autism?* Everyday Health. https://www.everydayhealth.com/aspergers/how-aspergers-different-than-autism/

Mattei, M. (2020, June 11). *Autism and Sleep - Patterns and Disorders Explained.* Sleep Advisor. https://www.sleepadvisor.org/autism-and-sleep/

Mayo Clinic Staff. (2018, January 6). *Autism spectrum disorder - Symptoms and causes.* Mayo Clinic; Mayo Foundation for Medical Education and Research. https://www.mayoclinic.org/diseases-conditions/autism-spec trum-disorder/symptoms-causes/syc-20352928

Meyers, M. (2016, January 31). *How Parents Can Help Their Autistic Children Make Friends.* WeHaveKids. https://wehavekids.com/parenting/How-to-Help-Your-Child-With-Autism-Develop-Meaningful-Friendships

Morin, A. (2022, September 4). *The Most Effective Ways to Discipline a Child With Autism.* Verywell Family. https://www.verywellfamily.com/disci pline-strategies-for-children-with-autism-4005045

Morrison, J. (2021, April 15). *5 Smart Ways to Identify Talent in an Autistic Child.* Mommy's Memorandum. https://mommysmemorandum.com/identify-talent-in-an-autistic-child/

Nedeoglo, K. (2019, June 21). *5 Steps to Leaving Your Autistic Child with a Caregiver.* Marvelously Set Apart. https://marvelouslysetapart.com/2019/06/21/autistic-child-with-caregiver/

Novak, S. (2022, December 2). *Autism Myths and Facts*. WebMD. https://www.webmd.com/brain/autism/features/autism-myths-facts

Obsessions - When is it Necessary to Correct Them? (2022, March 22). Healis Autism Centre. https://www.healisautism.com/post/obsessions-when-necessary-correct-them

Obsessions and repetitive behaviour - a guide for all audiences. (2020a, August 14). National Autistic Society. https://www.autism.org.uk/advice-and-guidance/topics/behaviour/obsessions/all-audiences

Obsessive Behaviour, Routines and Rituals: Autism Spectrum Disorder. (2021). Families for Life. https://familiesforlife.sg/parenting/Special-Needs/Pages/Development/Behaviour/Specialneeds_ASD_Obsessive_Routines_Rituals.aspx

Rice, A. (2021, September 6). *How Autism Affects Families: Challenges and Positives*. Psych Central. https://psychcentral.com/autism/how-autism-affects-family-life

Ryan, S. (2010). "Meltdowns", surveillance and managing emotions; going out with children with autism. *Health & Place, 16*(5), 868–875. https://doi.org/10.1016/j.healthplace.2010.04.012

Sarris, M. (2013, July 23). *Autism in the Teen Years: What to Expect, How to Help*. Interactive Autism Network at Kennedy Krieger Institute. https://www.kennedykrieger.org/stories/interactive-autism-network-ian/autism_in_teens

Sauer, M. (2016, April 1). *15 celebrity parents who've gotten real about raising kids with autism*. SheKnows. https://www.sheknows.com/parenting/slideshow/5643/celebs-who-have-kids-with-autism/4/

Seladi-Schulman, J. (2019, April 30). *Asperger's Treatment: Know Your Options*. Healthline Media. https://www.healthline.com/health/autism/aspergers-treatment

Siblings/Extended Family. (n.d.). Milestones Autism Resources. Retrieved April 19, 2023, from https://www.milestones.org/get-started/for-families/siblingsextended-family

Signs and Symptoms of Autism Spectrum Disorders. (2019a). Centers for Disease Control and Prevention. https://www.cdc.gov/ncbddd/autism/signs.html

Singer, E. (2010). The "W.I.S.E. Up!" tool: empowering adopted children to cope with questions and comments about adoption. *Pediatric Nursing, 36*(4), 209–212. https://pubmed.ncbi.nlm.nih.gov/20860261/

Singh, N. N., Lancioni, G. E., Karazsia, B. T., Myers, R. E., Hwang, Y.-S., & Anālayo, B. (2019). Effects of Mindfulness-Based Positive Behavior Support (MBPBS) Training Are Equally Beneficial for Mothers and Their Children With Autism Spectrum Disorder or With Intellectual Disabilities. *Frontiers in Psychology*, 10. https://doi.org/10.3389/fpsyg.2019.00385

Skibitsky, J. (n.d.). *Helping Children with Autism Grow into Productive Young Adults*. ABS Kids. Retrieved April 19, 2023, from https://blog.abskids. com/helping-children-with-autism-grow-into-productive-young-adults

Skoyles, C. (2018, October 8). *15 Successful People with Autism Who Have Inspired Millions of People*. Lifehack. https://www.lifehack.org/805825/ successful-people-with-autism

Sleep and autism. (2020b, August 20). National Autistic Society. https://www. autism.org.uk/advice-and-guidance/topics/physical-health/sleep/parents

Sleep problems and solutions: autistic children. (2020a, June 11). Raising Children Network Australia. https://raisingchildren.net.au/autism/health-wellbe ing/sleep/sleep-problems-children-with-asd

Smith, K. (2020, February 5). *Coping with Stress While Caring for a Child with Autism*. Psycom. https://www.psycom.net/coping-with-stress-while-caring-for-a-child-with-autism

Social skills for autistic children. (2023). Raising Children Network Australia. https://raisingchildren.net.au/autism/communicating-relationships/ connecting/social-skills-for-children-with-asd#helping-autistic-children-use-social-skills-in-different-situations-nav-title

Social Skills in Children with Asperger's Syndrome: Issues and Solutions. (2023b). Durham Region Autism Services. https://www.durham-autism.org/ social-skills-in-children-with-aspergers-syndrome/

Solomon, M., Iosif, A.-M., Reinhardt, V. P., Libero, L. E., Nordahl, C. W., Ozonoff, S., Rogers, S. J., & Amaral, D. G. (2017). What will my child's future hold? phenotypes of intellectual development in 2-8-year-olds with autism spectrum disorder. *Autism Research*, *11*(1), 121–132. https://doi. org/10.1002/aur.1884

Strategies to Address Repeated Verbal Phrases for Children. (2023). Watson Institute. https://www.thewatsoninstitute.org/watson-life-resources/situ ation/strategies-address-repeated-verbal-phrases/

Tatom, C. (2022, January 10). *Autistic Child Hitting Parents: Ideas and Solutions*.

Autism Parenting Magazine. https://www.autismparentingmagazine.com/child-hitting-parents-solutions/

Taylor, M. J., Gustafsson, P., Larsson, H., Gillberg, C., Lundström, S., & Lichstenstein, P. (2018). Examining the Association Between Autistic Traits and Atypical Sensory Reactivity: A Twin Study. *Journal of the American Academy of Child & Adolescent Psychiatry, 57*(2), 96–102. https://doi.org/10.1016/j.jaac.2017.11.019

The Autism Site. (2017, October 21). *8 Tips for Developing Patience with Your Child.* The Autism Site News. https://blog.theautismsite.greatergood.com/cs-patience-with-child/

Thriving as a Teenager with Autism: Top 5 Transition Tips! (2022, November 4). ABA Centers of America. https://www.abacenters.com/teenager-with-autism/

Tick, B., Bolton, P., Happé, F., Rutter, M., & Rijsdijk, F. (2016). Heritability of autism spectrum disorders: a meta-analysis of twin studies. *Journal of Child Psychology and Psychiatry, and Allied Disciplines, 57*(5), 585–595. https://doi.org/10.1111/jcpp.12499

Tobik, A. (2018). *Social Stories for Autistic Children.* Autism Parenting Magazine. https://www.autismparentingmagazine.com/social-stories-for-autistic-children/

Treatment and intervention services for autism spectrum disorder. (2019b, September 23). Centers for Disease Control and Prevention. https://www.cdc.gov/ncbddd/autism/treatment.html

Types of Sensory Issues in Autism. (2021, September 7). Behavioral Innovations - ABA Therapy for Kids with Autism. https://behavioral-innovations.com/blog/types-of-sensory-issues-in-autism-examples-and-treatment-options/

Uljarević, M., Prior, M. R., & Leekam, S. R. (2014). First evidence of sensory atypicality in mothers of children with Autism Spectrum Disorder (ASD). *Molecular Autism, 5*(1), 26. https://doi.org/10.1186/2040-2392-5-26

University of Rochester Medical Center. (2019). *Interacting with a Child Who Has Autism Spectrum Disorder.* Rochester.edu. https://www.urmc.rochester.edu/encyclopedia/content.aspx?contenttypeid=160&contentid=46

Vijayalakshmi, S., & Kripa, K. G. (2015, April). *Autism-Heavy Metal Toxicity and Herbal Remedies: A Review.* Research Gate. https://www.researchgate.net/

publication/275272100_Autism-Heavy_Metal_Toxicity_and_Herbal_Remedies_A_Review

Voight, D. (n.d.). *Link Between Autism and Mercury*. Denise Voight. Retrieved April 23, 2023, from https://www.denisevoight.com/blog/link-between-asd-and-mercury-toxicity

Watson, S. (2008, July). *Helping Your Child With Autism Get a Good Night's Sleep*. WebMD. https://www.webmd.com/brain/autism/helping-your-child-with-autism-get-a-good-nights-sleep

What should I do if my child with autism hits me? (2021, February 25). Therapeutic Pathways. https://www.tpathways.org/faqs/what-should-i-do-if-my-child-with-autism-hits-me/

Why Do Autistics Have Issues with Social Skills? (2017, August 8). AppliedBehaviorAnalysisEdu.org. https://www.appliedbehavioranalysisedu.org/why-do-autistics-have-issues-with-social-skills/

IMAGE REFERENCES

CDC. (n.d.). Pediatric Developmental Screening Flowchart. [Image]. Centers for Disease Control and Prevention. https://www.cdc.gov/ncbddd/autism/images/Screening-Chart-575x715.jpg?_=58552?noicon

Milton Keynes UK
Ingram Content Group UK Ltd.
UKHW020907080324
439029UK00015BA/857